Developmental Care
of the
Premature Baby

Developmental Care
of the
Premature Baby

JEANINE YOUNG
BSc (Hons), RGN, RM, Dip ANC,
ENB 405 and 998

Sebastian Diamond Mother & Baby Sleep Physiology
Laboratory, Department of Child Health, University of Bristol,
Bristol, BS2 8EG, UK

Baillière Tindall
London Philadelphia Toronto Sydney Tokyo

Baillière Tindall   24–28 Oval Road
London NW1 7DX

The Curtis Center
Independence Square West
Philadelphia, PA 19106–3399, USA

Harcourt Brace & Company
55 Horner Avenue
Toronto, Ontario, M8Z 4X6, Canada

Harcourt Brace & Company, Australia
30–52 Smidmore Street
Marrickville
NSW 2204, Australia

Harcourt Brace & Company, Japan
Ichibancho Central Building
22–1 Ichibancho
Chiyoda-ku, Tokyo 102, Japan

A catalogue record for this book is available from the British Library

ISBN 0–7020–2137–7

Typeset by WestKey Limited, Falmouth, Cornwall
Printed and bound in Great Britain by WBC Book Manufacturers,
Mid Glamorgan

Contents

Foreword

The enormous improvements in neonatal and perinatal care over the past three decades has led to the survival of ever increasing numbers of infants born after shorter and shorter gestation. This improved outlook has focused attention on the special needs during infancy and childhood of these tiny survivors. Although this improved survival has not, in general, led to increased numbers of infants surviving with major disabilities, the numbers of infants with such disabilities has certainly not decreased.

Whilst part of the improved survival of preterm infants has undoubtedly come from the careful application of the observations of physiologists and basic scientists, much has also come from the observations and experiences of those directly involved in the care of these infants. The importance of the environment in which the preterm infant is nursed was appreciated by Pierre Boudin almost 100 years ago and has been periodically 'rediscovered' at intervals throughout this century.

The experiences and observations of nurses and doctors who care for preterm infants have given anecdotal support for the importance of individualized baby-centred care planning within the neonatal intensive care unit. Such approaches certainly make the neonatal intensive care unit a more human, responsive and less-threatening environment for parents, staff and, most importantly, for babies.

The work reviewed in this book allows us to take this concept further—the environment in which the infant is cared for, and the approach to that care, may have measurable benefits to the baby in both the short and long term. A pleasant calm environment in which the baby is not subjected to loud noises, bright lights, or unexpected frequent physical assaults may not only be kinder and more humane, but may actually offer significant neurodevelopmental advantages to the baby.

The importance of this book is that it draws attention to the considerable volume of work which has been done in this area and allows the pratitioner of newborn care (whether nurse or doctor) to recognize the increasing evidence that a tiny preterm infant is more than the sum total of its collected physiological systems. The complexity of the neuro-developmental processes occuring in these tiny infants, and our limited ability to understand those processes, should remind us of the importance of considering the baby's needs, 'expectations', and abilities in all aspects of care.

The author of this book has considerable experience of the intensive care of critically ill infants which is used in ensuring that the evidence and recommendations are kept within a very practical persepective achievable in the busiest and most understaffed of neonatal intensive care units.

Professor Peter J Fleming
*Professor of Infant Health and Developmental Physiology,
Department of Child Health, Unversity of Bristol,
Bristol BS2 8BJ*

Preface

ADVANCES in the technical care of neonates have enabled smaller premature infants to survive (Becker *et al.*, 1991; Oehler, 1993; Stewart Hegedus and Madden, 1994), however neurodevelopmental sequelae continue to be a major source of morbidity (Barb and Lemons, 1989; MacPhee and Mori, 1991). It has been suggested that injury to the preterm developing brain resulting from the stressful nature of the intensive care environment is responsible for a portion of this overall morbidity (Als, 1986; Avery and Glass, 1989; Becker *et al.*, 1991; Gardner Cole *et al.*, 1990; Klaus, 1976; Oehler, 1993; Shultz, 1992; Vandenberg, 1985; White-Traut and Hutchens Pate, 1987).

Neonatal nurses, the primary caretakers in the special care baby unit, are in key positions to significantly and positively influence the environment of the developing neonate.

Utilizing a neurodevelopmental systems framework this book provides a critical analysis of recent literature relating to developmentally supportive care for preterm babies. The areas addressed focus on those which identify nursing care issues that affect the development of preterm infants: lighting, noise, handling, tactile or kinesthetic stimulation, massage and positioning.

Recommendations drawn from analysis of relevant literature in each area comprise a developmental care protocol for the nursing of preterm infants in the neonatal intensive care unit. The guidelines presented form a resource base which may assist neonatal nurses to develop individualized plans of care based on the assessment of each infant's behavioural cues, their response to environmental stimuli and care-giving interventions.

The ultimate goal of these intervention strategies in the neonatal intensive care unit is to facilitate and promote infant growth and development, and thus task mastery/performance (Korner, 1990; Merenstein and Gardner, 1993).

Utilization of developmental interventions in several American neonatal nurseries resulted in significant improvements in outcome, as demonstrated by a reduced number of days on assisted ventilation, earlier feeding success, shorter hospital stay, a marked reduction in number of complications and improved neurodevelopmental outcomes during the first 18 months of life (Als *et al.*, 1986; Becker *et al.*, 1991; Grunwald and Becker, 1991).

Successful implementation of developmental care protocols based on the recommendations proposed in this book may enable neonatal nurses throughout the UK to share these significant outcome improvements with their American colleagues and to improve the developmental outcome for premature infants in their care.

Acknowledgements

My sincere appreciation and thanks are expressed to the following people who offered support and encouragement throughout the compilation of this book.

Mr Bernard Place, for advice, encouragement and endless enthusiasm.

Ms Vivien Young, for sharing her knowledge and expertise in the area of supportive positioning for premature infants.

Dr Michael Bird, for his patience and support.

Miss Sarah Godeck, colleague, dear friend and empathetic listener.

Captain Alan and Mrs Sue Young, whose love and encouragement across the miles made all the difference.

Special thanks are expressed to Sarah and Boyden Manns, parents of Blair, a baby boy born at 28 weeks' gestation with a birth weight of 570 grams. Their unfailing commitment to the implementation of interventions that had the potential to enhance Blair's progress and development, and their ability to *know* their son and respond appropriately to his behavioural cues, clearly demonstrated to me that developmental care is achievable in practice.

It is to them that this book is dedicated.

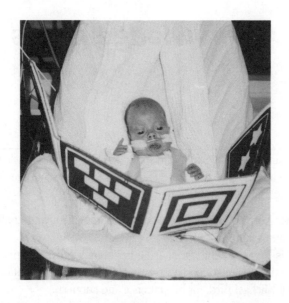

Blair Manns. Blair was born at 28 weeks' gestation, weighing only 540 grams. This picture (sitting up in the chair with a material book in front of him) was taken at 14 weeks of age (post birth date). He was discharged home on low flow oxygen after spending the first 26 weeks and 3 days of his life in hospital.

CHAPTER ONE

Introduction

SURVIVAL rates for infants born prematurely have improved over the past decade, but minimal advancement has been made in optimizing neurodevelopmental outcome (Barb and Lemons, 1989; Becker *et al.*, 1991; Lawhon and Melzar, 1988; Lipsi *et al.*, 1991; MacPhee and Mori, 1991; Oehler, 1993). Neurodevelopment is defined as 'the early development of neonatal neurological systems in relation to normal developmental patterns' (Shultz, 1992, p. 11).

Premature infants are accepted to be at significant risk of social, cognitive, linguistic and behavioural disturbances (Becker *et al.*, 1991; Shultz, 1992) and are also at risk for auditory, visual and neurodevelopmental deficits (Avery and Glass, 1989; Ellison, 1984). Even among infants with no apparent neurological or cognitive abnormality there is a relatively high incidence of deficits in information processing and attention-related disorders at preschool and school ages (McCormick, 1989). There is consensus in the literature (Als, 1986; Avery and Glass, 1989; Becker *et al.*, 1991; Gardner Cole *et al.*, 1990; Lynch, 1991; Oehler, 1993; Shultz, 1992; Vandenberg, 1985; White-Traut and Hutchens Pate, 1987) that a portion of this overall morbidity may represent injury to the developing brain resulting from the stressful nature of the intensive care environment. The relationships between fetal brain development, behavioural organization and the environment are examined briefly in Appendix A.

Harmful effects of care-giving

The vulnerability of the preterm baby is evident from the many deleterious effects associated with such 'routine' care interventions as handling, repositioning, oral and tracheal suction, weighing, radiographic examination and relocating monitoring probes (Peters, 1992). Physiological and behavioural reactions of distress during these interventions include apnoea (Gorski *et al.*, 1983; Murdoch and Darlow, 1984; Peters, 1992), hypoxaemia (Barnes and Kirchhoff, 1986; Danford *et al.*, 1983; Long *et al.*, 1980b; Peters, 1992; Speidel, 1978), cyanosis (Gardner Cole *et al.*, 1990), bradycardia and tachycardia (Gorski *et al.*, 1990; Fanconi and Duc, 1987; Murdoch and Darlow, 1984; Peters, 1992; Simbruner *et al.*, 1981), systemic hypertension (Fanconi and Duc, 1987), raised intracranial pressure (Perlman and Volpe, 1983), hyperexcitability (Gorski, 1985; Gorski *et al.*, 1983), states of arousal and activity (Gorski *et al.*, 1983; Gardner Cole *et al.*, 1990), vomiting (Gorski, 1985; Gorski *et al.*, 1983; Oehler *et al.*, 1991) and gasping (Gorski *et al.*, 1983).

Rather than too much or too little stimulation, it is now proposed that infants in the neonatal intensive care unit (NICU) receive an inappropriate *pattern* of stimulation, e.g. non-contingent, non-reciprocal, painful (rather than pleasant) and multiple stimuli (Blanchard, 1991; Gottfried and Gaiter, 1985; Heriza and Sweeney, 1990; Merenstein and Gardner, 1993). Recent research has shown medical and developmental benefits to preterm infants who receive individualized behavioural and environmental care (Als, 1986, Als *et al.*, 1986; Becker *et al.*, 1991; Grunwald and Becker, 1991).

Role of the neonatal nurse

Neonatal nurses, the primary caretakers in the special care baby unit (SCBU), are in a key position significantly and positively to influence the environment of the developing neonate (Wright Lott, 1989), and in accordance with the United Kingdom Central Council's *Code of Professional Conduct* (UKCC, 1992, p. 2) should 'ensure that no act or omission on his/her part or within his/her sphere of influence is detrimental to the condition or safety of patients' and 'take every reasonable opportunity to maintain and improve professional knowledge and competence'.

To fulfil their role, neonatal nurses must take responsibility for identifying and reducing stimuli in the preterm infant's environment which may damage the developing nervous system (Langer, 1990; MacPhee and Mori, 1991; Oehler, 1993; Tucker Catlett and Holditch-Davis, 1990). It is crucial to recognize that they can enhance the outcome of the preterm population by understanding their special physical needs, by possessing knowledge of neuromotor development, early intervention and parent education, and by interacting with interdisciplinary healthcare professionals (Campbell, 1986; Lynch, 1991; MacPhee and Mori, 1991).

Developmental intervention

The purpose of developmental intervention is twofold: (1) to reduce detrimental stimuli to the lowest possible level; and (2) to provide appropriate opportunities for development (Als, 1986;

Table 1.1 *Purpose of developmental intervention*

- To reduce detrimental stimuli
- To provide appropriate opportunities for development

Gorski, 1985; Gunderson and Kenner, 1987; Vandenberg, 1985; Whitley and Cowan, 1991; Wright Lott, 1989) (Table 1.1). Meeting both purposes of developmental care in a typical SCBU presents a tremendous challenge.

Using a neurodevelopmental systems approach this book critically reviews relevant literature, summarizes issues and puts forward recommendations for intervention in the developmental care of preterm infants. Systems discussed include the visual system, the auditory system, the somatosensory system and neuromotor development.

Implementation of developmental care in the intensive care nursery will be addressed through methods of assessing preterm behavioural cues and the formulation of a developmental care protocol for preterm infants based on the recommendations proposed after critical analysis of the literature. Finally, the potential impact of implementing such a developmental care protocol on the outcome for these preterm infants will be discussed.

CHAPTER TWO

Methods

Literature search

RESEARCH reports on developmental care for preterm neonates were reviewed using CINAHL and MEDLINE literature searches, published from January 1982 to August 1994 and from January 1989 to December 1993 respectively. Keywords used in the searches were 'preterm', 'developmental', 'handling', 'touch', 'positioning', 'massage', 'noise', 'light' and 'environment'. Reference lists were also obtained from a study day on 'Developmental Care in the Special Care Baby Unit: The NIDCAP Approach' held at St Mary's Hospital, London, in June 1994 and from personal communication with an American developmental specialist and researcher, Kathleen Vandenberg, who was guest speaker at this study day. Several research reports that were found to recur on reference lists of review articles obtained through the initial computer search were traced to their primary sources and added to this literature review.

Categorization of articles

The 131 relevant research reports and literature reviews obtained in this search of nursing, medical, physiotherapy, occupational therapy and developmental specialist sources have been grouped into the following broad categories which address preterm infants in the intensive care nursery. The number of articles addressing each category identified is included in parentheses. The categories include noise (4), lighting (7), reports addressing both noise and lighting (4), handling (16), positioning (24), touch/tactile stimulation (19), massage (11), kangaroo-care (9), factors contributing to intraventricular haemorrhage (7), behavioural assessment techniques (4), and developmental intervention strategies (26).

Without exception, the 26 articles that specifically address developmental care and intervention in this search were from the USA, and probably contributes to the fact that developmental care protocols have not yet been formulated and implemented, nor have further research findings been disseminated, to neonatal intensive care units (NICUs) in the UK.

Neurodevelopmental systems framework

For the purpose of this book, categories to be analysed focus on those that identify nursing care issues affecting the development of preterm infants; they have been organized into a neurodevelopmental systems framework (Table 2.1). Categories to be critically reviewed within each system are: light (visual system); noise (auditory system); handling, tactile or kinesthetic stimulation, and massage (somatosensory system); and positioning (neuromotor development). Discussion of systems in this sequence facilitates a progression from general environmental considerations, light and noise, to more specific care-giving

Table 2.1 *Neurodevelopmental systems framework*

- Visual system
- Auditory system
- Somatosensory system
- Neuromotor development

interventions involving handling and positioning. These are all factors potentially affecting the preterm infant in the NICU. Table 2.2 lists references found in each category, subdivided into literature reviews and empirical studies.

Light

Of the literature specifically addressing light, four empirical studies from both nursing (Blackburn and Patteson, 1991; Gordon Shogan and Schumann, 1993) and medical (Glass *et al.*, 1985; Mann *et al.*, 1986) sources were found. Each of these studies was chosen for critical analysis as, although in some instances different variables were measured, all were comparable in assessing the effects of lowering environmental lighting (Glass *et al.*, 1985; Gordon Shogan and Schumann, 1993) or of cycling light levels (Blackburn and Patteson, 1991; Mann *et al.*, 1986) may have on the preterm infant in the intensive care nursery.

Noise

Noise levels in the neonatal intensive care nursery have received intermittent attention in the paediatric literature (Long *et al.*, 1980a); most studies were carried out in the 1970s. This literature search yielded seven articles addressing noise (see Table 2.2), only two of which were empirical studies specifically investigating the effects of noise on infants in the intensive care nursery (Long *et al.*, 1980a; Strauch *et al.*, 1993). Additional research by

Horsley (1990) measured levels of noise, light and handling which neonates were exposed to in a 24-hour period, but did not assess physiological or behavioural effects on the infants. Although there appears to be a lack of recent definitive documentation of the long-term effects of special care baby unit (SCBU) noise on the preterm infant (Lotas, 1992), this does not mean that the effect of noise on the infant cannot be demonstrated. For this reason the study by Long and colleagues (1980a) has been included for analysis despite being over 10 years old, together with a nursing study by Strauch *et al.* (1993) addressing the effects of noise levels on infant sleep states, although neither study examined the preterm population exclusively.

Handling

Of information sources on handling of newborns requiring intensive care, 11 were empirical studies (see Table 2.2). Research for critical analysis was reduced by eliminating medical studies older than 10 years (Danford *et al.*, 1983; Gorski *et al.*, 1983; Long *et al.*, 1980b; Murdoch and Darlow, 1984; Speidel, 1978), all of which addressed the effects of handling on hypoxaemia. This effect was investigated in a more recent empirical nursing study by Cooper Evans (1991) and is included here for critical review. Remaining research studies for review are grouped into investigations in preterm infants of type of care-giver contacts (Werner and Conway, 1990), physiological responses to caregiver interventions (Cooper Evans, 1991; Gorski *et al.*, 1990; Peters, 1992) and behavioural and physical responses to developmental interventions during handling (McCain, 1992; White-Traut *et al.*, 1993). Responses of preterm infants to handling are well represented in both nursing and medical literature, although no evaluative studies for minimal handling protocols which have been proposed (Langer, 1990) were found during the search.

Tactile/kinesthetic stimulation and massage

The term 'tactile or kinesthetic stimulation' has also been referred to as 'stroking' or 'massage' in the literature (Field *et al.*, 1987); thus studies relating to both subjects have been reviewed together for the purpose of this book. Literature for analysis was selected from the 13 empirical studies available (see Table 2.2) on the basis that the research was less than 10 years old and the sample group was composed exclusively of preterm infants. In part, all the investigators in the five studies selected asked the research question: 'What effect does tactile/kinesthetic stimulation have on preterm infants?' (Adamson-Macedo, 1986; Blanchard *et al.*, 1991; Field *et al.*, 1986, 1987; Nelson *et al.*, 1986). An interesting observation was that information comprising this category was predominantly of nursing origin, which may reflect the growing recognition that nurses have a key role as primary care providers in investigating interventions that may enhance the outcome for preterm infants in the SCBU.

Positioning

A combined review of medical, physiotherapy and nursing research identified four key areas when considering correct positioning for premature infants; however, evaluative studies on the impact of positioning on preterm infant development were relatively limited. The key areas addressed were the effects of supine *versus* prone positioning on oxygenation and energy expenditure (Fox and Molesky, 1990; Lioy and Maginello, 1988; Masterson *et al.*, 1987), lateral positioning (Bozynski *et al.*, 1988), shoulder development (Georgieff and Bernbaum, 1986), cranial moulding (Alley, 1981; Budreau, 1987; Cartlidge and Rutter,

Table 2.2 *Literature of identified categories subdivided into review articles and empirical studies*

Category	Review	Empirical study
Noise	Letko (1992) (N)	Leonard (1993) (N) Long *et al.* (1980a) (M) Strauch *et al.* (1993) (N)

Light	Gardner and
	    Hagedorn (1990) (N)
	Glass (1993) (M)
	Sisson (1985) (M)
		Blackburn and Patteson
		    (1991) (N)
		Glass *et al.* (1985) (M)
		Gordon Shogan and
		    Schumann (1993) (N)
		Mann *et al.* (1986) (M)

Noise and light	Lotas (1992) (N) Treas (1993) (N) Weibley (1989) (N)	Horsley (1990) (N)

Handling	Field (1990) (M)
	Gunderson and Kenner
	    (1987) (N)
	Langer (1990) (N)
	Parker (1990) (N)
	Sparshott (1991) (N)
		Cooper Evans (1991) (N)
		Danford *et al.* (1983) (M)
		Gorski *et al.* (1983) (M)
		Gorski *et al.* (1990) (M)
		Long *et al.* (1980b) (M)
		McCain (1992) (N)
		Murdoch and Darlow
		    (1984) (M)
		Peters (1992) (N)
		Speidel (1978) (M)
		Werner and Conway
		    (1990) (N)
		White-Traut *et al.* (1993) (N)

Tactile/kinesthetic
stimulation
	Adamson-Macedo
	    (1990) (M)
	Barnett (1972) (N)
	Carruthers (1992) (N)
	Degen Horowitz
	    (1990) (M)
		Adamson-Macedo
		    (1986) (M)
		Blanchard *et al.* (1991) (P)
		Bodolf Rausch (1981)
		Field *et al.* (1986) (N)
		Harrison *et al.* (1990) (N)

Category	Review	Empirical study
	Ingham (1989) (N)	Harrison *et al.* (1991) (N)
	Korner (1990) (M)	Koniak-Griffin and
	Lester and Tronick	Ludington-Hoe (1988) (N)
	(1990) (M)	Nelson *et al.* (1986) (N)
	Sayre-Adams (1991) (N)	
	Slusher and McClure	
	(1992) (N)	
	Sparshott (1990) (N)	
	Tronick *et al.* (1990) (M)	
Massage		
	Adamson (1993) (N)	Booth *et al.* (1985) (N)
	Clarke (1992) (AT)	Field *et al.* (1987) (N)
	Isherwood (1994) (N)	Hartelius and Rasmussen
	Paterson (1990) (N)	(1992) (N)
	Russell (1993) (N)	White-Traut and Goldman
	Weber (1991) (AT)	(1988) (N)
		White-Traut and
		Hutchens Pate (1987) (N)
Positioning		
	Bellefeuille-Reid and	Alley (1981) (M)
	Jakubek (1989) (O)	Bozynski *et al.* (1988) (M)
	Bottos and Stefani	Budreau (1987) (N)
	(1982) (M)	Cartlidge and Rutter
	Cubby (1991) (N)	(1988) (M)
	Elmer and Gregg	Downs *et al.* (1991) (P)
	(1979) (M)	Fox and Molesky (1990) (N)
	Fay (1988) (N)	Georgieff and
	Munro (1988) (M)	Bernbaum (1986) (M)
	Perez-Woods *et al.*	Hemingway and Oliver
	(1992) (N)	(1991) (N)
	Pym (1992) (P)	Kurlak *et al.* (1994) (N)
	Turrill (1992) (N)	Lioy and Maginello (1988) (M)
	Updike *et al.* (1986) (O)	Marsden (1980) (M)
	Warren (1993) (N)	Masterson *et al.* (1987) (M)
	Young (1994) (N)	

Letters in parentheses denote the source of information: N, nursing; M.
medical; P, physiotherapy; O, occupational therapy; AT, alternative therapy.

Table 2.3 *Analysis of research studies in developmental care*

Purpose of study	Setting	Subject sample	Experimental conditions
LIGHTING Gordon Shogan and Schumann (1993) examined the relationship between environmental illumination and oxygen saturation in premature infants.	Tertiary NICU	n=27, convenience sample of caucasian preterm infants, 26–37 weeks' gestation. *Criteria for inclusion*: > 2 days of age Normal haematocrit and haemoglobin values Free from sepsis No phototherapy No maternal diabetes Informed parental consent	Infants served as their own controls. All monitored with head at 20° angle, in prone position, during interval between scheduled feeding or treatments and while sleeping. Procedure: 1) Room illuminance measured with overhead lights on. 2) S_aO_2 data collected continuously for 5 min to establish baseline. 3) At 5 min overhead lights dimmed, incubator covered, illumination measured. 4) S_aO_2 measured at 1 and 5 min and continuously over 30 min. 5) After 30 min, lights returned to previous illumination levels; incubator uncovered. S_aO_2 recorded 1 and 5 min after lights increased. Any intervening variables occurring during study period, e.g. loud noises, were recorded.
Blackburn and Patteson (1991) examined the effects of different lighting conditions on activity state and cardiorespiratory function in preterm infants.	Tertiary NICU	n=18, convenience sample of 18 preterm infants born < 34 weeks' gestation. No history of major anomalies or maternal drug addiction	*Continuous light group* (n=9) No attempt was made to control when lights were turned off or on for these infants. *Cycled light group* (n=9) Overhead and individual lights were turned off for a portion of the 24-hour period. OFF: during evening (from 1600 to 0026 hours) ON: in morning (from 0600 to 0900 hours) Lights were turned on briefly every 2–3 hours for care-giving during lights-off.

Data collection	Analysis	Results	Limitations
Oxygen saturation data collected continuously from Nellcor oximeter N2000, using a Nellcor N9000 analog strip chart recorder. Investigator timed procedural intervals.	Descriptive analysis – (mean and standard deviation). Repeated measures analysis of variance (ANCOVA). χ^2 analysis.	No significant difference found in oxygen saturation after decreasing light; 22% of infants had clinically significant S_aO_2 reduction within 1 min after lights increased. *Conclusion:* Rapid increase of environmental light from 5 to 100 foot-candles may be a stressor for babies who are gestationally and postnatally younger.	Infants may have habituated to the 100 foot-candles baseline light levels in the NICU, which may have affected the results of decreasing the lights. Small sample size. Possible compromise of internal validity with intervening variable, as environmental noise was not controlled and was noted to have an effect.
Time-lapse video recordings of infant activity and lighting conditions. Cardiorespiratory data via Hewlett-Packard monitor was synchronized with video using internal computer–clock and time–date generator. Infant activity coded using an eight-point scale.	Experimental design. ?t test analysis to test differences between statistical measures of two samples.	Heart rate and activity were lower in cycled group than for 'lights on' group. No difference in respiratory rate noted. Longer periods of inactivity and quiescence in cycled lighting group. *Conclusion:* Decreasing light levels during evening and night may facilitate rest and subsequent energy conservation in preterm infants.	Changes in heart rate and activity may be related to overall environmental changes rather than to reduced lighting, i.e. when lights are dimmed, noise and staff activity are also reduced; possible compromise of internal validity. Infants allocated to subject groups and method used to analyse or compare data were not reported. Small sample size. Parental consent not reported.

Table 2.3 *Continued*

Purpose of study	Setting	Subject sample	Experimental conditions
NOISE Long *et al.* (1980a) examined: (a) ambient noise levels before and after modification or elimination of noise-producing activities; and (b) the effects of noise on a preterm infant's behaviour and physiological response.	Tertiary NICU	(a) NICU staff and environment. (b) *n*=2, male preterm infants, 7 days old: (i) 35 weeks' gestation, 2430 g, no supplemental oxygen (ii) 34 weeks' gestation, 2020g, incubator oxygen at 25%	(a) *Environment* *Control period*: Baseline noise levels, measured in decibels (dB). Measurements taken at various positions in the nursery between 0800 and 1500 hours; five 3-hour recordings taken over 1 week. *Test period*: Following modification of greatest noise-producing machines and discussion re reducing noise-producing activities with staff, the above procedure was repeated together with levels taken within incubators. (b) *Infants* Infants served as their own controls. Over a 2-hour period sound levels, heart rate (HR), respiratory rate (RR), transcutaneous partial pressure of oxygen $P_{tc}O_2$) and intracranial pressure (ICP) were monitored.
Strauch *et al.* (1993) examined the effect of a quiet hour protocol on noise levels and infant sleep states.	Newborn developmental unit (NDU)	Admission criteria NDU: Levels 1 and 2: minor to prolonged developmental disruptions requiring limited to defined intervention to facilitate normal development and prevent or ameliorate physical and psychosocial effects. Level 3: severe or chronic problem requiring structured intervention to facilitate normal function at their potential. Level 4: infant whose death is imminent (within 24 hours) for whom no heroic measures are planned.	*Control observations*: Noise levels and infant state measured for 1 week. *Quiet hour protocol:* Implemented for 3 weeks for 1 hour at end of each 8-hour shift. Weeks 1 and 2: routine established. Week 3: noise levels and infant state measured. *Quiet hour protocol:* 1) Reduce talking to a whisper at bedside 2) Allow no large equipment to enter unit 3) Make special effort not to slam doors, trash cans, incubator doors or drag chairs. 4) Permit no physician rounds 5) Respond rapidly to alarms and crying infants 6) Forward all phone calls to the desk 7) Rearrange care-giving activities to minimize infant disturbance

Data collection	Analysis	Results	Limitations
(a) *Environment*: Noise measured with general radio 1565-A sound level meter set to A-weighted scale, calibrated to multi-pen chart recorder for continuous recording. (b) *Infants*: 4 hours of polygraphic recordings made of HR, RR, $P_{tc}O_2$ and ICP. ICP measured via anterior fontanelle using Ladd ICP monitor.	(a) Strict quantitative analysis not performed. Comparisons made of high-amplitude deflections to activities of staff. Records from control and test periods compared. (b) No statistical analysis evident. Polygraphic recording of one infant supplied.	Baseline noise levels 60–65 dB. All high-amplitude recordings associated with staff activity. Reduced baseline dB, frequency and height of deflections during test period. *Conclusion*: NICU staff contribute to ambient noise level. Decrease in $P_{tc}O_2$ and increases in HR, RR and ICP observed in response to noise stimuli. *Conclusion*: Noise may be a cause of hypoxaemia.	External validity questionable — study sample of infants limited. Requires replication with larger sample and/or multicentre trial. Experimental conditions did not limit possible intervening variables, e.g. handling, light, to account for hypoxaemia. No statistical analysis; descriptive comparisons only.
Noise levels: monitored by handheld decibel meter in five locations in unit; collected during last hour of each 8-hour shift, for 7 consecutive days. *Infant state*: as described by Als (1983, cited by Strauch *et al.*, 1993), measured by trained raters; inter-rater reliability 0.90.	*Noise levels*: by $5 \times 3 \times 7 \times 2$ analysis of variance (location x shift x day x trial) with shift nested within location and repeated measures of last two factors. *Infant state*: analysed by Kruskal–Wallis test on effect of trial, day or shift (control *versus* quiet hour) on infant state.	Mean noise levels were higher midweek (64 dB) than over weekends (52 dB), with a significant decrease in noise during the quiet hour (52.2 dB) compared with control levels (58.3 dB). Infants spent more time in deep or light sleep during quiet hour periods. *Conclusion*: Noise levels in NDUs can be significantly decreased by means of an intervention period of noise reduction, and reduced noise levels have a positive effect on infant state.	Subjects not necessarily the same in each control or intervention phase, and randomization of infants was not possible. Potential for confounding events between data collection periods. Number of infants participating in study not reported. Number of interruptions during quiet hour not measured. No control for infant development or severity of illness.

Table 2.3 *Continued*

Purpose of study	Setting	Subject sample	Experimental conditions
HANDLING AND TOUCH Cooper Evans (1991) examined (a) frequency, (b) duration and (c) magnitude of hypoxaemic episodes related to care-giving activities during the first 72 hours of life for preterm infants with RDS, and (d) identified activities associated with the greatest decreases in $P_{tc}O_2$	Tertiary NICU	n=13, convenience sample of preterm infants. *Criteria for inclusion*: Diagnosis of RDS < 34 weeks' gestation < 72 hours of age Normal haematocrit, haemoglobin and temperature Appropriate size for gestational age No congenital abnormality Intubated and on intermittent ventilation	*Definitions* *Caregiving activities*: Intervention involving tactile contact between care-giver and infant or attached equipment. *Hypoxaemia*: $P_{tc}O_2$ < 50 mmHg for over 1 min *Hyperoxaemic*: $P_{tc}O_2$ > 100 mmHg for over 1 min *Control period*: *period*: minimum of 10 min rest before observation period. *Observation period*: Physiological data ($P_{tc}O_2$, HR, RR and BP) continuously recorded for 60 min; colour and activity documented by researcher every minute; no attempt made to control type or sequence of care-giving interventions. Observer changed every 30 min to prevent fatigue.
Field *et al.* (1987) examined the effects of massage on preterm infant growth and development.	Tertiary NICU to 'grower nursery'	n=40 *Criteria for inclusion*: Medically stable < 36 weeks' gestation < 1500 g birth weight No congenital heart malformations, CNS disturbances, drug addictions or congenital anomalies No supplemental oxygen or intravenous feedings All infants nursed in isolette and bottle-fed	*Control group*: n=20; no controlled tactile stimulation period. *Treatment group*: n=20; tactile stimulation delivered for three 15-min periods at beginning of three consecutive hours, 30 min after first morning feed for 10 week-days (weekend excluded). Stimulation sessions: three standardized 5-min phases. Phases 1 and 3: tactile stimulation—stroking in prone position. Phase 2: kinesthetic stimulation—passive flexion and extension movements in supine position (timing and number of strokes detailed in Field *et al.* 1987). At end of treatment: sleep–wake behaviour observations recorded for 45 min

Data collection	Analysis	Results	Limitations
Novametrix 818 Transcutaneous Oxygen monitor provided continuous monitoring printout of $P_{tc}O_2$. Dynograph R611 physiological chart recorder provided continuous form printouts of HR, RR and BP. Anderson State/Activity Scale used to code infant activity on a scale of 1–12.	Planimetred means calculated for control period of each recording. Descriptive statistics used to determine frequency of hypoxaemia and time taken to return to baseline. Frequency counts of interventions with evaluation of associated $P_{tc}O_2$ changes.	Care-giving was provided for mean of 24% of observation period (range 6–26 min). Most frequent activities were suctioning, repositioning and sampling for blood gas analysis. Hypoxaemic episodes: 0–3 per infant; mean 6.8 min per episode or 11.3 min per infant. Mean magnitude of $PtcO_2$ decreased 39.7 mmHg. *Conclusion:* Handling and care-giving activities may cause hypoxaemia.	Infants did not all receive the same care-giving procedures, limiting interpretation of results. No control over type or sequencing of interventions. Intervening variables, e.g. noise and light, may have contributed to results, thus a threat to internal validity of study. Small sample size. Parental consent not reported. No control for severity or instability of infant illness; threat to internal validity.
Clinical data recorded from hospital charts, i.e. weight, number and volume of feeds. Brazelton Neonatal Behaviour Assessment Scale administered at end of treatment period. Inter-rater reliability 90%. Sleep–wake behaviour recorded via nine-point coding system in 10-s intervals. Inter-rater reliability 85%. 6 month follow-up: growth measures and Bayley Scales of Infant Development.	Multivariate and univariate t tests to determine how stimulation affected treatment of infants.	Stimulated infants averaged 47% greater weight gain per day; at 6-month follow-up, improved performance on Brazelton habituation, orientation, motor and range of state items; more active during sleep–wake observations; improved performance on Bayley Mental and Motor Scales compared with control infants. *Conclusion:* Tactile stimulation appears to facilitate growth and development of preterm infants.	Severity of neonatal illness and home environment is known to influence outcome, but not reported in sample description. Bayley Scales of Infant Development are a poor predictor of cognitive outcome. Method used to calculate inter-rater reliability not reported.

Table 2.3 *Continued*

Purpose of study	Setting	Subject sample	Experimental conditions
POSITIONING Fox and Molesky (1990) examined the relationship between PaO_2 and supine or prone positions in neonates with RDS.	Tertiary NICU	n=25, preterm neonates. *Criteria for inclusion:* ≤ 36 weeks' gestation Diagnosis of RDS Endotracheal intubation and intermittent mandatory ventilation and/or continuous positive airway pressure Receiving supplemental oxygen Functional umbilical artery oxygen tension catheter *in situ* Not receiving paralysing drugs Informed parental consent obtained	Infants nursed in incubator, on baffled water beds with head of bed elevated 30°. Each infant to be observed in prone and supine positions, thus each baby served as its own control. Random assignment of first position to be recorded by coin toss. *Procedure*: Position 1, infant allowed to settle to sleep before data collection. P_aO_2 measurements began a minimum of 5 min after positioning (range 5–19 min) and continued every 30 s for 15 min. Infant then turned to position 2, allowed to settle and the procedure was repeated. Data collected within a 1-hour period, during which ventilatory and oxygen parameters remained unchanged. Descriptions of prone and supine positions provided.
Downs *et al.* (1991) examined whether maintaining functional postures during hospital admission prevents development of the frog-lying or flattened posture.	Tertiary NICU	n=45, convenience sample of preterm infants. *Criteria for inclusion:* < 33 weeks' gestation Parental consent obtained No genetic or congenital limb anomalies	Random number table used to assign groups. *Control group:* n=24; infants positioned according to usual nursing practice for the neonatal unit. The prone position without hip support was favoured. *Treatment group*: n=21; specific hip support, commencing at 7 days of age and continuing until the baby was at least a corrected age of 36 weeks, was provided for the intervention group. *Prone*: positioned with pelvic elevation, bearing weight through anterior knee, and hips not flexed >90. *Sidelying*: trunk supported perpendicular to surface with both arms forward; bottom leg in neutral position. *Supine*: knees and elbows supported off surface to reduce hip and shoulder abduction.

Data collection	Analysis	Results	Limitations
Arterial P_aO_2 measured via an indwelling electrode in the umbilical artery oxygen tension catheter and attached to Neocath 1000 monitor to give continuous readout of oxygen pressure after calibration with actual arterial blood gas samples (checked before data collection to ensure accurate calibration).	Two-tailed paired t test: P_aO_2 for prone positioning compared with that for supine positioning	Mean P_aO_2 for infants in the prone position was 71.5 mmHg compared with 65.2 mmHg for the supine position ($t = 3.72$, $P = 0.005$) *Conclusion:* Prone positioning of the intubated neonate with RDS results in significantly higher P_aO_2 than does supine positioning.	Sample restricted to intubated preterm infants with RDS. Results may not apply to term infants, to infants with other conditions, or to those without endotracheal tubes and positive pressure ventilation. Infants were nursed on baffled water beds that placed less pressure on the abdomen than may be achieved on different water beds or mattresses. Subjects were all studied in deep sleep to minimize the effect of state on P_aO_2. It is unknown whether differences in PaO_2 between the two positions would have been maintained if the subjects had been studied for longer than 15 min.
Positioning implemented and supervised by neonatal physiotherapist. Postural assessment performed on infants at mean gestational plus postnatal age 40 (range 36–42) weeks by paediatricians. *Pronelying:* weight-bearing surface of lower limb observed. *Sidelying:* if position was maintained independently, recorded as stable; if not, recorded as unstable; *Supported standing:* deviation from position of neutral rotation measured.	χ^2 analysis with Yates' correction to analyse prone and sidelying positions. Mann–Whitney U test to analyse angles of total external leg rotation in the supported position.	More infants in intervention group lay taking weight through anterior aspect of knee, were able to maintain sidelying independently, and had a lower angle of external hip rotation than those in the control group. *Conclusion:* Specific hip support during the period of intensive care results in fewer features of abnormal posture at the equivalent of term.	Interobserver reliability for 40-week postural assessment stated in study as 'checked'; however, method used to determine value and the actual value calculated were not reported. Some infants were discharged home before postural assessment at a mean of 40 (range 37–44) weeks. Home environment is a sociodemographic variable known to influence outcome, but not reported in the sample description.

BP, blood pressure; CNS, central nervous system; HR, heart rate; ICP, intracranial pressure; NDU, newborn developmental unit; NICU, neonatal intensive care unit; P_aO_2, arterial partial pressure of oxygen; $P_{tc}O_2$, transcutaneous partial pressure of oxygen; RDS, respiratory distress syndrome; RR, respiratory rate; SaO$_2$, oxygen saturation.

1988; Hemingway and Oliver, 1991; Marsden, 1980) and hip posture (Downs *et al.*, 1991). Five studies from this research with results that have direct implications for guiding clinical nursing practice were chosen for critical review (Downs *et al.*, 1991; Fox and Molesky, 1990; Georgieff and Bernbaum, 1986; Hemingway and Oliver, 1991; Masterson *et al.*, 1987).

Analysis of studies

Research questions posed in the empirical studies selected for critical analysis are listed together with data relating to the various instruments, statistical analyses, findings and limitations in Table 2.3. Tabular analysis facilitated closer examination and comparison of sample groups and of the methodology used in studies addressing the same neurodevelopmental system, and the identification of research questions requiring further investigation and validation. Recommendations for nursing intervention are proposed following analysis in the critical review.

CHAPTER THREE

The Visual System

Effects of light on the preterm infant

THE VISUAL system is the last sensory system of the central nervous system (CNS) to develop and is therefore the most immature at birth (Als, 1986; Oehler, 1993). Lighting in most neonatal intensive care units (NICUs) is continuous, high level and fluorescent (Jorgensen, 1993; Tucker Catlett and Holditch-Davis, 1990), with the intensity of light increasing five to tenfold over the past two decades (Glass *et al*, 1985; Gordon Shogan and Schumann, 1993; Wolke, 1987). There is now growing concern about the consequences of this exposure to light in premature infants, who may spend weeks or even months in an intensive care nursery (Glass *et al.*, 1985; Jorgensen, 1993; Oehler, 1993).

The effects of light on the premature infant are emerging in research focusing on four main questions:

1 What light patterns and intensity are common to the NICU?
2 What are the effects of lighting levels on the development of retinopathy of prematurity (ROP) and other visual impairments?

3 What are the effects of lighting on the infant's physiological responses and development?
4 What are the effects of lighting patterns and day–night cycles on the functioning of the infant?

Illumination levels

A survey of illumination levels of NICUs in the UK reported mean levels of approximately 24–90 foot-candles (approximately 240–900 lux) (Robinson *et al.*, 1990), while other studies have proposed light intensity in the NICU averages 60–80 foot-candles (ft-c) (Blackburn and Patteson, 1991; Oehler, 1993; Wolke, 1987) (refer to the Glossary for a definition of illumination units). Peak light exposure for the infant was found to be associated with additional light sources such as heat lamps (200–300 ft-c) (Blackburn and Patteson, 1991; Lotas, 1992), phototherapy lamps (300–400 ft-c) (Blackburn and Patteson, 1991; Glass *et al.*, 1985; Lotas, 1992) and, most dramatically, extensive direct window exposure supplementing artificial lighting (levels of 1000 ft-c) (Gordon Shogan and Schumann, 1993; Lotas, 1992; Oehler, 1993). This is in contrast to the recommendation of 40–50 ft-c for regular office lighting by the Occupational Safety and Health Administration in the USA (Gordon Shogan and Schumann, 1993; Lotas, 1992; Oehler, 1993) and the most recent *Guidelines for Perinatal Care* published by the American Academy of Pediatrics (1992), which state that 60 ft-c is recommended in the NICU for adequate observation and 100 ft-c for procedures (Table 3.1).

Infants' eyes are routinely protected during phototherapy (Fig. 3.1), but not while they are under a heat lamp or near a window (Glass *et al.*, 1985). For many years, continuous lighting was considered to be necessary for surveillance of all infants in intensive and intermediate care nurseries; however, with

Table 3.1 *Recommendations for light levels in the NICU*

- 60 ft-c for adequate observation
- 100 ft-c for procedures

Source: American Academy of Pediatricians, 1992

advanced monitoring capabilities it is now proposed that many infants do not require continuous bright lighting (Blackburn and Patteson, 1991; Gottfried and Gaiter, 1985; Yecco, 1993).

Retinal damage

A causative link between exposure to continuous bright lighting and damage to the retina of the premature infant has not yet been conclusively established. Early animal studies using a primate model (Messner *et al.*, 1978; Moseley and Fielder, 1988; Sykes *et al.*, 1981; all cited by Lotas, 1992) documented retinal damage secondary to short periods of intense lighting, which

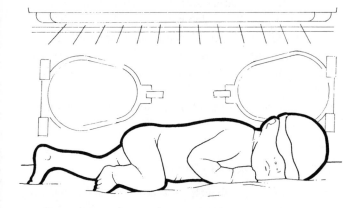

Figure 3.1 *Example of an eye shield used to protect an infant's eyes during phototherapy.*

was greater with continuous than with cycled light (Kramer and Pierpoint, 1976, cited by Oehler, 1993). Although these studies are suggestive and demonstrate significant retinal damage at light levels reported in the NICU environment (400–500 ft-c), they should be interpreted with caution as they did not study the lower light levels more common in the nursery or the effects of long-term exposure such as a premature infant would be likely to experience (Lotas, 1992; Treas, 1993).

Investigations by Glass *et al.* (1985) demonstrated a 32% increased incidence of ROP in a group of infants (n=74) exposed to the brighter nursery lights (median 60 ft-c) than in those (n=154) for whom light levels were reduced (median 25 ft-c), particularly in infants with birth weights below 1000 g. A serendipitous finding in this study was that 76% of infants in the protected group who developed ROP were in incubators placed by a window, and who thus experienced periodic exposure to light intensitites in excess of 400 ft-c. However, a similar study by Ackerman and colleagues (1989, cited by Lotas, 1992; Oehler, 1993) with a larger sample group of 290 infants did not find a significant relationship between ROP and brighter nursery lights (55 ft-c *versus* 15 ft-c), and these results relating environmental lighting to ROP have not been replicated (Treas, 1993). In summary, studies examining the relationship between nursery lighting levels and ROP are inconclusive and preliminary at best, but do support the need to continue this line of investigation.

Other physiological effects

In addition to concern about the effects of light on the premature visual system, investigations into the effects of NICU lighting on other aspects of the infant's physiological and behavioural functions have begun. Studies of the effects on humans show that intense, cool, white light causes chromosomal damage (Treas, 1993) and changes in biological rhythms (Oehler, 1993; Tucker Catlett and Holditch-Davis, 1990), endocrine gland and gonadal function (Gordon Shogan and Schumann, 1993; Gottfried and Gaiter, 1985; Yecco, 1993), and vitamin D synthesis (Treas, 1993; Yecco, 1993). Studies by Clyman and Rudolph (1978, cited by Lotas, 1992) and Rosenfeld *et al.* (1986, cited by Oehler, 1993) also suggest a relationship between excessive lighting from phototherapy and the incidence of patent ductus arteriosus.

Oxygen saturation

Nurse researchers, Gordon Shogan and Schumann (1993), investigated the relationship between environmental illumination and oxygen saturation in preterm neonates. This was the only study found in the literature search which addressed immediate infant responses to changes in illumination and was chosen for analysis as its results and recommendations have implications for neonatal nursing practice.

In a convenience sample of preterm infants ($n=27$), oxygen saturation data were collected continuously via non-invasive oximetry, a method easily observed by nurses (Gordon Shogan and Schumann, 1993). A comprehensive description of the experimental procedure was provided, together with statistical methods used in data analysis (see Table 2.3), although measures of interobserver reliability, which may affect treatment integrity (Thomas and Conway, 1992), were not mentioned in the report.

Results demonstrated no significant difference in oxygen saturation after lights were reduced. The researchers considered the possibility that the infants had become habituated to the 100-ft-c baseline levels in the NICU to account for this result. However, 22% of infants experienced a clinically significant drop in oxygen saturation within 1 min after the light intensity was increased. The researchers concluded that a rapid increase in environmental light from 5 to 100 ft-c may be a stressor for babies who are gestationally and postnatally younger, although a decrease in environmental lighting may not improve oxygen saturation in the majority of infants.

This study employed strict selection criteria and had subjects serve as their own controls which, although removing many of the threats to internal validity (Thomas and Conway, 1992), also reduces the number of possible subjects in a small population — a common problem in neonatal research (Dyke and Conway, 1992), and one recognized by the researchers. Replication in a multicentre study may increase external validity if similar results are obtained in different settings (Thomas and Conway, 1991). Environmental noise was not controlled, which may have served as an intervening variable to compromise the internal validity of the study (Thomas and Conway, 1992). These limitations were acknowledged by the researchers in their recommendations for similar studies in a noise-free environment and with a larger sample group requiring oxygen and ventilatory assistance.

This study has implications for neonatal nursing practice. In an NICU, rapidly returning lights to levels of 100 ft-c after such procedures as echocardiography (ECG) and ultrasonography, which require near darkness to facilitate better visualization, may cause some infants, especially those gestationally and postnatally younger, to desaturate. Placing lights on rheostats which gradually increase and decrease the intensity of the light may moderate this response. This study demonstrates how preterm infants must be observed and cared for individually, which concurs with the findings of Als (1986) that preterm infants have a better outcome when each neonate is individually assessed and a specific plan of care initiated.

Effects of lighting patterns

The fourth area of research related to NICU lighting comes from the growing number of studies examining the effects of light–dark cycles on physiological functions, and the development of sleep–wake patterns and circadian rhythms. Exposure of pre-term infants to day–night patterns has been reported to increase time spent sleeping (Blackburn and Patteson, 1991; Mann *et al.*, 1986; Sheldon and Bell, 1987, cited by Lotas, 1992; Weibley, 1989), to decrease motor activity and heart rate (Blackburn and Patteson, 1991; Shiroiwa *et al.*, 1986, cited by Lotas, 1992; Oehler, 1993), to decrease fluctuations in blood pressure (Blackburn and Patteson, 1991; Mann *et al.*, 1986), to increase eye opening and duration of alert state (Moseley *et al.*, 1988, cited by Oehler 1993), to reduce feeding time (Jorgensen, 1993; Mann *et al.*, 1986), to increase weight gain in medically stable infants (Blackburn and Patteson, 1991; Jorgensen, 1993; Mann *et al.*, 1986; Weibley, 1989) and to result in earlier synchronization of the infant's behavioural and hormonal rhythms with the external environment (Jorgensen, 1993; Sisson, 1985). These findings suggest improved behavioural organization (Lotas, 1992; Oehler, 1993).

A study by Blackburn and Patteson (1991) examined the effects of different lighting conditions on activity state and cardiorespiratory function, and was selected for further analysis as the results of the study have implications for clinical practice (see Table 2.3). Data were collected from 18 preterm infants via time-lapse video recordings and cardiorespiratory monitoring equipment. Selection criteria were provided, with no significant differences found between the infants assigned to the cycled lighting group (lights turned off for a portion of the 24-hour day) (*n*=9) and those who experienced continuous lighting conditions (*n*=9).

Results suggest that reduced heart rates, with longer periods of inactivity and quiescence similar to quiet sleep, are achieved when lights are cycled for premature infants. No significant differences were noted in respiratory rate. The researchers concluded that decreasing light levels during the evening and night may facilitate rest and subsequent energy conservation in preterm infants.

The study has several limitations. No reference was made to proxy consent given by parents, which raises legal and ethical issues (Holditch-Davis and Conway, 1992; Treas, 1993), and methods used to analyse data were not specified, although it appears a *t* test analysis was used to test significant differences between statistical measures of the two samples (Oehler and Cusson, 1994). Changes in heart rate and activity may also have been related to overall environmental changes, i.e. it was noted that when lights were dimmed staff activity and noise were also reduced, which may compromise the internal validity of the study (Thomas and Conway, 1992). A threat to treatment integrity was identified when the researchers stated that, because this was a naturalistic study, no attempt was made to control when the lights were turned off and on for each infant in the continuous light group; these decisions were made by the infant's nurse. This may have led to diffusion of the treatment into the control group, as described by Thomas and Conway (1992): raised awareness of the treatment, in this case the lowering of lights, leads nurses caring for the control groups also to use the treatment. External validity would be enhanced by replications of the study using a larger sample group or in a multicentre trial (Thomas and Conway, 1991).

Recommendations for clinical practice

The review of literature highlights several issues for clinical practice. The most basic observation is that light levels in NICUs are often intense and demonstrate little diurnal variability. Although inconclusive, there is some evidence to suggest that damage to the visual system occurs with exposure to excessive lighting, and several studies have demonstrated improvements in behaviour with reduced and cycled light.

Given the lack of evidence for any benefits of bright lighting, it would be a prudent approach in the NICU to reduce ambient light to levels necessary to observe the infant and monitoring equipment safely, and to shield the eyes from ambient as well as supplementary sources (Glass, 1993; Lotas, 1992; Oehler, 1993). Shielding, however, does not mean occluding the infant's eyes, as there is no evidence to support the usefulness of patching the infant's eyes beyond what is necessary for phototherapy (Glass, 1993). The American Academy of Pediatrics (1992) recommends 60 ft-c for adequate observation; 100 ft-c is sufficient for procedures.

Practical modifications

Modification of lighting in NICUs may by implemented in various ways. Overhead lighting can be reduced by use of dimmer switches (Blackburn and Patteson, 1991; Gordon Shogan and Schumann, 1993; Lotas, 1992); lights can be turned off when not in use (Lotas, 1992; Oehler, 1993); and individual lights can be used when additional lighting is needed for procedures (Lotas, 1992; Whitley and Cowan, 1991). Curtains or window shades can be used to reduce sunlight levels (Blackburn and Patteson, 1991; Lotas, 1992; Whitley and Cowan, 1991). Infant Developmental Care Guidelines by the National Association of Neonatal Nurses

(NANN) (1993, cited by Treas, 1993) support nursing interventions of dimming room lights and covering incubators and cribs to minimize exogenous stressors of ambient room light and noise. Potential benefits of covering the incubator include reduction of ambient light; reduction of noise through a padded interface; availability of diurnal variation; insulation of the incubator; and provision of a physical barrier to remind caregivers to allow periods of uninterrupted rest (Treas, 1993).

Covering infants in incubators, radiant warmers and cribs with a blanket, quilt or other material, e.g. empty nappy boxes, reduces infant exposure to bright overhead lights or daylight, and are methods employed in units throughout the USA (Blackburn and Patteson, 1991; Treas, 1993; Tucker Catlett and Holditch-Davis, 1990; Whitley and Cowan, 1991). A commercially prepared incubator cover has been designed with adjustable flaps to allow care-giver visibility, with the fabric selected to permit accurate evaluation of skin colour (Treas, 1993) (Fig. 3.2). However, these techniques are rarely used with acutely ill infants because the cover prevents the nurse directly observing the infant's condition. Tucker Catlett and Holditch-Davis (1990) suggest a small drape placed over the headbox or arranged in a tent-like fashion over the infant's head and neck, if assisted ventilation is necessary. This drape provides visual darkness for the ill infant while allowing staff adequate visualization of fingers, toes and trunk.

Safe practice

The issue of the negative sequelae of environmental illumination on the premature infant has been addressed in litigation proceedings. Parents have filed suits because their infant developed ROP when the incubator was not covered despite numerous studies documenting the potential negative effects of exposure

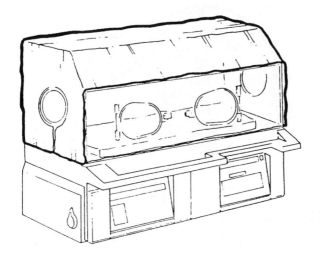

Figure 3.2 *Incubator covers minimize oxogenous stressors of ambient light and noise.*

to bright lights (Treas, 1993). On the other hand, the risk of litigation is high if harm comes to the infant as a result of the care-giver's inability to visualize a problem, e.g. a kinked endotracheal tube. It appears the care-giver is in a precarious position.

Nurses are responsible for providing reasonable and prudent care (Lynch, 1991). After review of the literature available, and in the name of patient safety, the author recommends that an unobstructed view of the critically ill infant is provided while ambient room light is reduced at intervals throughout the day and night, a view supported by Treas (1993). For the stable preterm infant, a drape partially covering the incubator or crib to block excessive light, while allowing assessment of infant colour, positioning and equipment (Fig. 3.3), is an intervention supported in the literature (Barb and Lemons, 1989; Whitley and

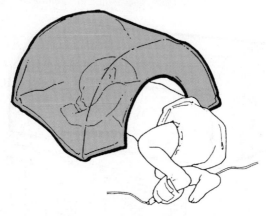

Figure 3.3 *A drape partially covering a headbox. An infant's colour, positioning and equipment may still be safely observed while using a drape to reduce excessive light.*

Cowan, 1991; Yecco, 1993). Recommendations for controlling environmental light have been included in the Protocol for Developmental Care of the Premature Infant (Appendix B).

CHAPTER FOUR

The Auditory System

Effects of noise on the preterm infant

NOISE levels in the neonatal intensive care unit (NICU) are a major source of environmental stress for premature infants (Long *et al.*, 1980a; Lotas, 1992; Oehler, 1993; Treas, 1993; Tucker Catlett and Holditch-Davis, 1990; Whitley and Cowan, 1991). Studies examining the effects of NICU auditory stimuli on the premature infant have focused on four general questions:

1. What is the quantity and quality of sound in the NICU?
2. What are the sources of that sound?
3. Is there any interactive effect with any of the ototoxic drugs used for the neonate?
4. Can any alteration in infant function or developmental outcome be documented in association with either the quality and/or quantity of NICU sound?

Noise levels

Researchers have repeatedly documented sound levels of 50–90 decibels (dB) in the NICU (Horsley, 1990; Jorgensen, 1993; Letko,

1992; Long *et al.*, 1980a; Lotas, 1992; Oehler, 1993; Strauch *et al.*, 1993; Weibley, 1989), comparable to light traffic and light machinery respectively (Lotas, 1992; Oehler, 1993), with peaks recorded as high as 120 dB (Jorgensen, 1993; Lotas, 1992). The Occupational Safety and Health Administration in the USA describes 90 dB as the highest sound-safe level for adults, with no safe levels developed as yet for infants and children (Lotas, 1992; Oehler, 1993). In an ordinary home an infant is usually exposed to 40 dB (Oehler, 1993). In addition, NICU noise levels demonstrate little diurnal variation and few fluctuations. When they occur, they do so in an unpredictable manner (Lotas, 1992).

Much of the sound present in the NICU is generated by the equipment used to care for infants, including incubators, oxygen monitoring devices, ventilators and infusion pumps (Lotas, 1992; Oehler, 1993; Weibley, 1989), with centrifuges, monitor alarms and telephones contributing significantly to the high-amplitude sound recordings (Lotas, 1992; Weibley, 1989). Less anticipated findings, reported by Long *et al.* (1980a), were that most high-amplitude sounds, 70 dB or more, were related to staff activities, including laughter, conversation, and the closing of doors, garbage lids, incubator ports and drawers (Fig. 4.1).

The incubator is also poor protection from environmental sound (Fig. 4.2). Studies have shown noise levels in incubators to be identical to those in the room (Gottfried and Gaiter, 1985; Horsley, 1990; Oehler, 1993), with harsh mechanical noises clearly penetrating the isolette (Yecco, 1993), in addition to the constant noise of the incubator motor and fan at average levels of 60–75 dB (Oehler, 1993; Yecco, 1993).

Causes of hearing loss

Although it has not yet been possible to prove a direct causative effect of noise on hearing loss, owing to confounding variables

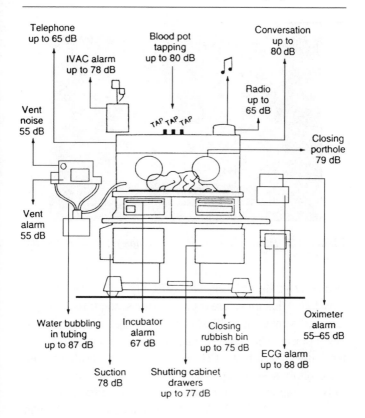

Figure 4.1 *Environmental noise and the premature infant. The recommended mean noise level inside the incubator is 60 dB. Adapted from a poster by Bernadette Brewster, with permission.*

such as hyperbilirubinaemia and the use of aminoglycoside antibiotics (Letko, 1992; Lotas, 1992; Oehler, 1993), premature infants experience hearing loss at a rate of 13% compared with 2% among term infants (Letko, 1992; Shultz, 1992).

Animal studies (Barnard and Pechere, 1984; Gannon *et al.*, 1979; cited by Lotas, 1992; and Bhattacharyya *et al.*, 1986;

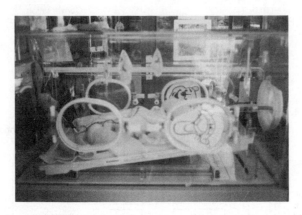

Figure 4.2 *The incubator is poor protection from environmental sound.*

Dodson *et al.*, 1982; Douek *et al.*, 1976; all cited by Oehler, 1993) have found that immature organisms are susceptible to temporary and permanent cochlear damage during critical periods of development, when receiving aminoglycosides and exposed to incubator noise. Infants of 24–26 weeks' gestation are born when the auditory system is maturing and are therefore more likely to be susceptible to the combined effects of drugs and noise (Letko, 1992; Oehler, 1993). Although no studies of human neonates have documented the occurrence of an interactive effect between ototoxic drugs and NICU noise (Lotas, 1992; Oehler, 1993), in view of findings from animal experimentation, concern about such an effect remains reasonable.

Other effects of environmental noise

Short and long-term outcomes for the premature infant resulting from environmental noise were examined by the final group of studies. Long *et al.* (1980a) examined the immediate responses of infants to noise following a quantitative assessment of sound and its sources in the NICU (see Table 2.3). This study was limited by a small sample of premature infants ($n=2$) and absence of statistical analysis other than comparison of polygraphic recordings of the two infants, but a repeated pattern of decreased transcutaneous oxygen tension and increased intracranial pressure, heart and respiratory rates were documented in response to sudden loud noises in the nursery.

The conclusion that noise may cause hypoxaemia, indicative of an infant stress response, was supported in later studies reporting mottling, apnoea and bradycardia (Gagnon, 1989, cited by Jorgensen, 1993; Gottfried and Gaiter, 1985; Gorski *et al.*, 1983) and decreases in transcutaneous partial pressure of oxygen ($P_{tc}O_2$) of 10 or more points (Holditch-Davis and Thoman, 1987, cited by Oehler, 1993) in preterm infants exposed to sharp sound incursions. These studies suggest that NICU noise levels are a disorganizing influence on the neurologically immature infant and raise questions regarding the energy cost of these episodes to the infant (Lotas, 1992).

Another concern identified was the potential detrimental effect of noise on the infant's processing of auditory stimuli (Lotas, 1992; Oehler, 1993; Yecco, 1993). The continuous nature of ventilator and incubator sounds, together with unexpected loud noises of alarms or people laughing (Letko, 1992; Tucker Catlett and Holditch-Davis, 1990), combined with the effect of containing an infant in an incubator which deflects sound, including the human voice (Yecco, 1993), may cause 'disjunctive stimulation' (Oehler, 1993). The premature infant is not able to identify the origin of the sound, which may limit its opportunity to integrate multimodal aspects of the environment (Lotas, 1992; Oehler, 1993; Yecco, 1993).

The quiet hour protocol

Although there has been a lack of definitive documentation on long-term effects of NICU noise on the premature infant (Lotas, 1992), this area is beginning to be explored. Strauch and colleagues (1993) investigated the effect of a quiet hour on noise levels and sleep state of infants in a newborn developmental unit (NDU). Noise levels were monitored and infant sleep states measured before and during the implementation of a quiet hour protocol (described in Table 2.3). Conclusions drawn from this study suggest that overall noise levels can be significantly decreased with an established intervention period of noise reduction, and that, when noise levels and procedural interruptions are decreased, the sleep states of infants are enhanced.

Some limitations of this study must be noted. Several documented problems of pre–post design (Burns and Grove, 1993) were evident with this study. First, subjects were not necessarily the same in each control or intervention phase, as infants were selected by means of the location of their cribs; randomization of infants was not possible. Second, there was a potential for confounding events to occur between data collection periods. No efforts were made to control for infant development or severity of illness. However, infant turnover occurred during both periods of data collection, and infants were assigned to cribs for clinical reasons, without regard to the study. It was also possible that considerable variation in noise, interruptions and infant state occurred, as interruptions during the quiet hour were not measured, and infant state and noise levels were recorded only once during the last hour of each 8-hour shift.

The findings of this study should be regarded as preliminary in view of these limitations. Replication with controls for infant development and illness, and studies to investigate the impact of the quiet hour on physiological outcome and parental and staff stress levels, may assist in validating these findings in other NICUs and NDUs. None the less, this study has implications for clinical practice, demonstrating that some methods of reducing noise and interruptions are easily implemented by the nurse, and in this NDU, the study increased nurses' awareness of how noise may affect their patients, families and themselves (Strauch *et al.*, 1993).

Recommendations for clinical practice

A review of research related to the effect of NICU noise on the developing premature infant does not provide definitive evidence of long-term consequences. However, it does provide support for realistic concern and, until safe levels of noise are established (Oehler, 1993), justification for the modification of sound levels when possible (Horsley, 1990; Long *et al.*, 1980a; Lotas, 1992; Strauch *et al.*, 1993; Whitley and Cowan, 1991; Yecco, 1993). British Safety Standards (Table 4.1) require that mean noise levels inside an incubator should not exceed 60 dB (Horsley, 1990). However, many impact noise situations exceed this limit (Oehler, 1993; Strauch *et al.*, 1993; Yecco, 1993).

Ways to reduce sound levels

The following suggestions are made for reduction of sound in the NICU. Staff can begin to monitor activities such as talking and laughing; opening and closing doors, drawers and incubator ports; the manipulation of equipment; removing water from ventilator tubing; and responding quickly to monitor alarms or crying infants, to ensure that associated noise levels are kept to a minimum (Lotas, 1992; Strauch *et al.*, 1993; Whitley and Cowan, 1991). Care-givers and visitors could be encouraged to

Table 4.1 *British safety standards for incubator noise*

- Noise levels inside an incubator should not exceed 60 dB.

Source: British Safety Standards, Horsley 1990

conduct conversations away from the incubator or outside the care-giving area when possible (Strauch *et al.*, 1993; Whitley and Cowan, 1991; Yecco, 1993). Radios, intercoms and other extraneous sound could be eliminated from the NICU (Horsley, 1990; Lotas, 1992; Tucker Catlett and Holditch-Davis, 1990).

Equipment in the nursery could be modified when possible to reduce sound reaching the infant. Flashing lights could replace bells on telephones or they could be placed away from the care-giving area (Letko, 1992; Weibley, 1989); computer printers could be equipped with sound-proof covers (Lotas, 1992; Weibley, 1989); and the volume of monitor alarms could be reduced as practically as possible (Letko, 1992) or replaced by flashing alarms (Lotas, 1992; Strauch *et al.*, 1993).

Primary consideration should be given to noise levels generated when considering new or replacement equipment (Lotas, 1992; Weibley, 1989). Lotas (1992) advocates the use of carpeting and acoustic ceilings to reduce noise levels significantly in the NICU; however, the maintenance of infection control measures would have to be considered in the practical implementation of these proposals. In addition, covering the incubator with a padded interface is a nursing intervention supported by the NANN 1993 Infant Developmental Care Guidelines (Treas, 1993) to reduce ambient room noise reaching the infant.

The value of establishing a quiet period in the NICU is evident from studies that demonstrated overall reduced noise levels, enhanced infant sleep–wake patterns and reduced stress levels perceived by parents and staff (Blackburn and Patteson, 1991; Strauch *et al.*, 1993), while Vandenberg (1985) advocated posting

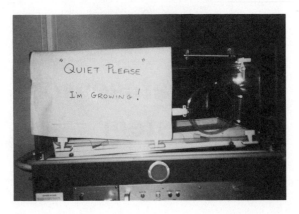

Figure 4.3 *'Quiet signs' may raise awareness of staff and parents to the preterm infant's need for noise level control.*

'quiet signs' by the cotside to raise staff and parent consciousness of the preterm infant's need for noise in the NICU to be controlled (Fig. 4.3).

Finally, the development of guidelines for acceptable noise levels should be established for the NICU to serve as a standard when selecting nursery equipment. This would also encourage manufacturers to design and develop quieter equipment for use in the NICU. Recommendations for reducing environmental noise are included in the Protocol for Developmental Care of the Premature Infant (Appendix B).

CHAPTER FIVE

The Somatosensory System

Effects of handling and tactile/kinesthetic stimulation on the preterm infant

PHYSICAL touch is the environmental stressor of premature infants over which nurses have the most control (Cooper Evans, 1991; Peters, 1992; Tucker Catlett and Holditch-Davis, 1990). Touch in the neonatal intensive care unit (NICU) primarily involves two forms: the uncomfortable or painful handling during nursing and medical procedures, and touch initiated for the purpose of social interaction (Tucker Catlett and Holditch-Davis, 1990; Yecco, 1993).

Procedural touch is a far more common phenomenon than social interaction (Whitley and Cowan, 1991; Yecco, 1993), and evidence suggests that, seemingly innocuous, routine procedures employed in the care of the preterm baby can have profound effects on the infant's condition (Cooper Evans, 1991;

Danford *et al.*, 1983; Gorski *et al.*, 1990; Long *et al.*, 1980b; Murdoch and Darlow, 1984; Peters, 1992; Speidel, 1978; Werner and Conway, 1990; White-Traut *et al.*, 1993). There is growing concern that most tactile stimulation is of poor quality for infant development (Tucker Catlett and Holditch-Davis, 1990).

Studies examining the effects of handling and care-giving procedures focus on two main questions:

1 What are the type, frequency and duration of care-giving contacts experienced by preterm infants in the NICU?
2 What physiological responses are demonstrated by preterm infants to care-giving interventions?

Type and amount of handling

In 1975, Korones (cited by Wolke, 1987) reported that observation of a group of 11 sick infants revealed a mean of 132 contacts over a 24-hour period. By 1984, the frequency was reported to be 40 to 70 with some infants receiving up to 100 contacts over 24 hours (Gottfried and Hodgman, 1984), with the mean duration of uninterrupted rest for each infant reported to be only 4.6–10.2 minutes (Duxbury *et al.*, 1984, cited by Werner and Conway, 1990).

A recent nursing study by Werner and Conway (1990) explored the type, frequency and duration of contacts experienced by ventilated preterm infants ($n=11$). A total of 645 contacts were made over 1210 minutes of observation. Treatment-oriented procedures accounted for 27.4% of contacts, while 63.7% were incidental, e.g. sound of incubator doors or accidental disturbance. Activities of daily living accounted for 4.5% and comfort measures only 4.4%. Nurses provided 82.6% of all contacts, consistent with finding of Korones (1984, cited by Wolke, 1987), with comfort measures provided primarily by parents.

Conclusions drawn suggest that premature infants whose basic need is to be at rest, are in fact subjected to high levels of tactile and auditory stimulation, consistent with previous findings which reported that some sick infants experience a mean of 100 (Gottfried and Hodgman, 1984) to 132 (Korones, 1975, cited by Wolke, 1987) contacts over a 24-hour period. These findings present a challenge to neonatal nurses to coordinate necessary care with comfort measures and to decrease the frequency of disruptive contacts with premature infants.

Infant distress from handling

A growing body of evidence from nursing and medical research indicates that any handling of critically ill or premature infants has the potential to cause distress (Cooper Evans, 1991; Gorski *et al.*, 1983; Long *et al.*, 1980b; Murdoch and Darlow, 1984; Norris *et al.*, 1982; Peters, 1992; Speidel, 1978). These negative physiological responses are reported to include apnoea (Gorski *et al.*, 1983; Murdoch and Darlow, 1984; Speidel, 1978); significant decreases in heart rate (Cooper Evans, 1991; Gorski *et al.*, 1983; Murdoch and Darlow, 1984; Speidel, 1978), transcutaneous oxygen tension (Cooper Evans, 1991; Danford *et al.*, 1983; Gorski *et al.*, 1983, 1990; Long *et al.*, 1980b; Murdoch and Darlow, 1984; Norris *et al.*, 1982; Peters, 1992; Speidel, 1978) and transcutaneous oxygen saturation levels (Peters, 1992); and significant increases in respiratory rate (Speidel, 1978), heart rate (Gorski *et al.*, 1983, 1990; Long *et al.*, 1980b; Peters, 1992; Speidel, 1978), blood pressure (Peters, 1992) and intracranial pressure (Gorski *et al.*, 1990; Peters, 1992). Frequent handling also disturbs sleep, leading to reduced weight gain and state regulation (Jorgensen, 1993; Wolke, 1987).

Hypoxaemia

Investigations by Cooper Evans (1991) examined the frequency, duration and magnitude of hypoxaemic episodes in preterm infants and identified the activities associated with the greatest decreases in oxygenation (see Table 2.3). Results indicated that care-giving was performed for a mean of 24% of the observation period (range 6–26 minutes per hour). The activities most frequently recorded were suctioning, repositioning and sampling for blood gas analysis, and were associated with the greatest decreases in transcutaneous partial pressure of oxygen ($P_{tc}O_2$), consistent with the findings of Norris *et al.* (1982). Other care-giving procedures identified in the literature (Danford *et al.*, 1983; Norris *et al.*, 1982; Speidel, 1978; Wolke, 1987) with a decrease in $P_{tc}O_2$ include chest radiography; physical examinations, phototherapy, chest physiotherapy, electrode changes, heel stabs, vital signs, weighing, tube and bottle feeding and diapering (Fig. 5.1); these observations were supported by Cooper Evans (1991). Hypoxaemic episodes ranged from 0 to 3 per infant with a mean of 6.8 minutes per episode (or 11.3 minutes per infant). The mean magnitude of reduction in $P_{tc}O_2$ was 39.7 mmHg, consistent with the findings of Speidel (1978), who reported a mean change of 31 mmHg in $P_{tc}O_2$ associated with care-giving procedures.

Apart from the small sample size, several threats to the internal validity of the Cooper Evans (1991) study may also limit interpretation of results (Thomas and Conway, 1992). Infants did not all receive the same care-giving procedures, thus the type and sequencing of interventions were not controlled; nor was there control for severity of infant illness. Intervening variables, e.g. light and noise, were not monitored, which may have contributed to the results for hypoxaemia associated with care-giving procedures.

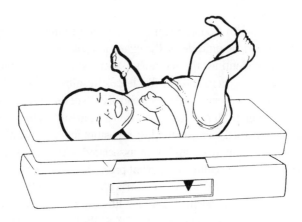

Figure 5.1 *Care-giving procedures such as weighing or blood sampling by heel stab may stress the preterm infant.*

Minimal handling

Despite these limitations, the investigator's conclusions have significant clinical implications. Handling and care-giving activities may cause hypoxaemia. Care-givers who are alert to infant stress signals may also be able to alter their pattern of care to eliminate or reduce episodes of associated hypoxia (Cooper Evans, 1991). These conclusions are supported by research (Gorski *et al.*, 1990; Langer, 1990; Long *et al.*, 1980b, Norris *et al.*, 1982; Speidel, 1978) which indicates that the timing of procedures may influence the infant's ability to recover. Clustering of care, although minimizing the number of times the incubator is opened and creating periods of rest between caretaking sessions, may cause a prolonged period of hypoxia and must therefore be individualized according to observed levels of infant tolerance (Langer, 1990). Peters (1992) also recommends that nurses should remain with the infant for 2–5 minutes after any procedure. Adverse responses to handling have occurred up to 5 minutes (range 0–300 seconds) after completion of care-giving, while the caretaker often leaves the cotside within 2 minutes of finishing the task (Peters, 1992).

Supplemental stimulation

Tactile and vestibular stimulation, it is suggested, provides continuity with the intrauterine environment (White-Traut and Goldman, 1988). Studies using tactile or kinesthetic stimulation have reported a variety of benefits, including improved performance on developmental tests (Field *et al.*, 1986, 1987), increased growth and weight gain (Field *et al.*, 1986; Whitley and Cowan, 1991), earlier discharge (Field *et al.*, 1986), reduced pain response by increasing endorphin production (Nelson *et al.*, 1986; Paterson, 1990), reduction of stress behaviours (Nelson *et al.*, 1986), possible facilitation of the sucking reflex (Adamson-Macedo, 1986) and promotion of parental bonding and attachment (Booth *et al.*, 1985; Harrison and Woods, 1991; Paterson, 1990; Russell, 1993; White-Traut and Hutchens Pate, 1987). Although indicating contradictory results for growth, with no differences in weight gain between stimulated and controlled infants, Blanchard and colleagues (1991) demonstrated that tactile stimulation in a controlled form did not cause hypoxaemia in their sample of preterm infants.

Field and colleagues (1987) used weight gain and developmental assessments to measure the effectiveness of a supplemental stimulation programme for 40 preterm infants (see Table 2.3). Each infant in the treatment group ($n=20$) received tactile/kinesthetic stimulation through a set delivery procedure for 10 days. Results indicated that stimulated infants averaged a 47% greater weight gain (mean of 8 g per day) inclusive of the 6-month follow-up; showed improved performance on the

Brazelton assessment at 10 days and on the Bayley mental and motor scales at 6 months; and were more active during sleep–wake observations. The investigator concluded that tactile stimulation for preterm infants appears to be a cost-effective form of facilitating growth and development.

However, several limitations are important to consider with this study. Severity of neonatal illness and home environment, neonatal and sociodemographic variables known to influence outcome (Page and Cusson, 1993), were not reported in the sample description and may have influenced follow-up results. The Bayley scales of infant development have also been demonstrated to be a poor predictor of infant cognitive outcome (Page and Cusson, 1993), thus the reliability and validity of some test measures used in the study are questionable.

It is important to note that all of the studies reviewed which examined tactile stimulation involved medically well, premature infants who did not require respiratory support. The safety of these procedures for younger, sicker infants has not been established (Oehler, 1993). In view of the negative effects of handling noted above and studies that have demonstrated negative effects even of social touching in high-risk infants (Harrison and Woods, 1991; Oehler, 1988, cited by Oehler, 1993), tactile stimulation should be approached cautiously in immature high-risk infants.

Pacification

Finally, the effects of environmental stimulation on acutely ill premature infants can be reduced by using pacification techniques—nursing interventions that reduce distress by calming the infant and promoting sleep. Several interventions, including containment of the infant's movement by swaddling (Tucker Catlett and Holditch-Davis, 1990), non-nutritive sucking (Oehler, 1993) and encouraging grasping behaviour (Whitley and Cowan,

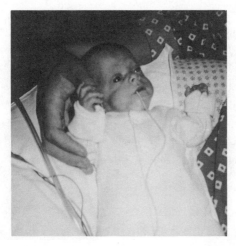

Figure 5.2 *Grasping behaviour can be used as a pacification technique to reduce distress by calming the infant and promoting sleep.*

1991) (Fig. 5.2), have been found to be effective, although their use may not be widespread at present.

Swaddling
Premature infants, who generally have a low threshold for stimulation and become irritable with overstimulation (Cooper Evans, 1991; Langer, 1990; Oehler, 1993), may be soothed by the warmth and security of swaddling (Fig. 5.3). Although the effects on premature infants have not been studied in detail, swaddling normal full-term infants has been reported to reduce crying and increase time spent asleep (Brackbill, 1971, cited by Tucker Catlett and Holditch-Davis, 1990; Romanko and Bost, 1982). Tucker Catlett and Holditch-Davis (1990) observed increases in transcutaneous oxygen levels of 15–25 mmHg after 10 minutes of swaddling in a group of premature infants. The

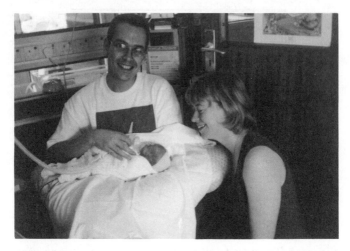

Figure 5.3 *Swaddling contains the infant's movements and reduces stress.*

same group of infants demonstrated heart rate decreases of 10–20 beats per minute, and a move from the stage of fussing to quiet alertness within 5 minutes of swaddling.

Non-nutritive sucking

Non-nutritive sucking, given in conjunction with gavage feedings and between feeds, has been associated with numerous positive outcomes for infants. The benefits include higher levels of oxygenation during gavage feedings (Nading and Landes, 1984; Pickler and Terrell, 1994) and at rest (Woodson *et al.*, 1985), decreased heart rate (Woodson and Hamilton, 1988), greater weight gain (Woodson *et al.*, 1985), accelerated maturation of sucking resulting in a faster transition from gavage to oral feeding (Bernbaum *et al.*, 1983; Sehgal *et al.*, 1990; Woodson *et al.*, 1985), increased levels of alertness before feedings (McCain,

1992) and earlier discharge home (Bernbaum *et al.*, 1983; Merenstein and Gardner, 1993; Sehgal *et al.*, 1990). These benefits have not been fully explained, although two possible explanations have been proposed.

It has been suggested that the improved weight gain, more rapid transition from gavage to oral feeding, and shorter hospital stay found with the use of non-nutritive sucking during gavage feedings are associated with enhanced gastrointestinal function. In particular, insulin secretion has been noted to increase when non-nutritive sucking is provided during gavage feedings (Marchini *et al.*, 1987, cited by Pickler and Terrell, 1994), which may improve glucose utilization. In addition, an increase in gastrin secretion and a decrease in somatostatin secretion have been reported when non-nutritive sucking is provided during gavage feeding (Widstrom *et al.*, 1988, cited by Pickler and Terrell, 1994). Gastrin secretion stimulates acid secretion, gastric motility and the growth of intestinal mucosa. Somatostatin inhibits gastric emptying; therefore reduced levels of this hormone should increase gastric transit. The mechanism responsible for these changes in enzyme and hormone levels is thought to be related to stimulation of the vagus nerve by sucking (Pickler and Terrell, 1994).

However, some studies have found no increase in gastric transit time when infants are given non-nutritive sucking during gavage feeding (De Curtis *et al.*, 1986; Szabo *et al.*, 1985). Other studies have also found no significant increase in gastric lipases levels (Smith *et al.*, 1987, cited by Pickler and Terrell, 1994), serum protein concentrations (Ernst *et al.*, 1989) or energy and fat absorption (De Curtis *et al.*, 1986), following treatment with non-nutritive sucking. Preliminary studies investigating the possible protective effect of non-nutritive sucking against the development of necrotizing enterocolitis are as yet inconclusive (Pickler and Terrell, 1994). Prospective studies of larger sample

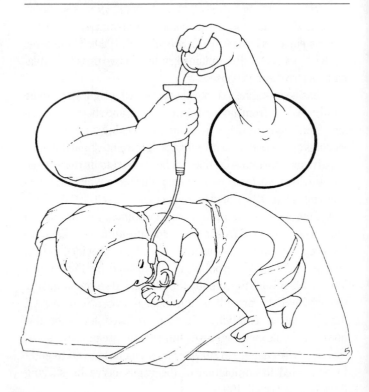

Figure 5.4 *Non-nutritive sucking during gavage feeding is associated with reduced energy expenditure and improved behavioural states.*

sizes that involve examination of the effect of non-nutritive sucking on gastric motility and enzyme and hormone secretion are needed.

A second explanation for the positive effects of non-nutritive sucking is related to optimal behaviour states associated with this intervention. Non-nutritive sucking has been demonstrated to reduce the time that preterm infants spend in active behaviour states, to increase the time spent in a quiescent behaviour state and to decrease the frequency of behaviour state changes (Compos, 1989; Di Pietro *et al.*, 1994; Field and Goldson, 1984). In addition, non-nutritive sucking provided before bottle feedings has been shown to reduce restless states and increase quiet alert states (McCain, 1992), while following bottle feedings it promotes a more rapid transition to a quiescent behaviour state (Di Pietro *et al.*, 1994; Pickler *et al.*, 1993).

Thus, non-nutritive sucking may be an effective modulator of behaviour state. The benefits associated with it may be related to the decrease in energy expenditure and improved neurobehavioural organization associated with the optimal behaviour states achieved (Fig. 5.4).

Recommendations for clinical practice

Long-term effects of care-giver interventions upon the behavioural organization of the extremely premature infant are not known (Oehler, 1993; Werner and Conway, 1990). It can only be assumed that stimuli inherent in the environment may create behavioural disorganization (Als, 1986; Vandenberg, 1985; Werner and Conway, 1990). Potentially negative effects may be reduced by nurses becoming more aware of behavioural and autonomic cues, and utilizing them in organizing the infant's care according to individual tolerance levels (Cooper Evans, 1991; Jorgensen, 1993; Shultz, 1992; Yecco, 1993).

Procedures to minimize handling

Interactions with infants should be coordinated to minimize handling and provide periods of uninterrupted rest (Jorgensen, 1993; Whitley and Cowan, 1991). Routine procedures should be evaluated for their necessity (Whitley and Cowan, 1991) and limited to essential procedures, particularly for babies requiring considerable support (Oehler, 1993). Routine vital signs can be taken from the monitor and checked by auscultation only once per shift (Tucker Catlett and Holditch-Davis, 1990).

Care-giving should be timed to cluster activities as tolerated by the infant, and time should be provided for recuperation and reorganization (Jorgensen, 1993; Langer, 1990; Oehler, 1993), which may help prevent intraventricular haemorrhage (Cooper Evans, 1991; Dietch, 1993; Kling, 1989). The very unstable infant may have difficulty tolerating any procedure, requiring a rest period between each intervention.

Techniques to prevent distress

Some units have developed 'hands off' times (Langer, 1990; Whitley and Cowan, 1991) during which all non-emergency procedures are postponed to assure infants an opportunity for undisturbed sleep (Fig. 5.5), and care is planned to coincide with the infant's awake or more alert periods (Cooper Evans, 1991; Lawhon and Melzar, 1988). Alerting techniques can be used to rouse an infant gently before a care-giving procedure to prevent startling (Lawhon and Melzar, 1988; Whitley and Cowan, 1991). Methods including swaddling (Oehler, 1993; Tucker Catlett and Holditch-Davis, 1990), offering non-nutritive sucking (Cooper Evans, 1991; Whitley and Cowan, 1991) and encouraging grasping (Lawhon and Melzar, 1988; Whitley and Cowan, 1991) have been used effectively to reduce motoric activity, oxy-haemoglobin desaturation and adverse responses, and assist in calming the infant during handling and unpleasant procedures (Langer, 1990; Oehler, 1993; Whitley and Cowan, 1991).

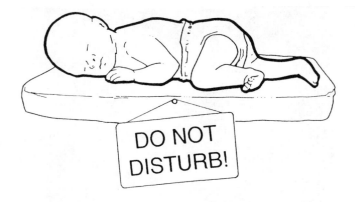

Figure 5.5 *'Hands Off' times assure the infant of opportunities for undisturbed sleep.*

Swaddling

Swaddling the premature infant in the NICU requires modification of traditional swaddling techniques. Tucker Catlett and Holditch-Davis (1990) advocated placing a blanket over the infant from the shoulder down and tucking its ends securely under the mattress, as the most effective method (Fig. 5.6). This technique provides motor restraint, increased warmth and easy access, if needed (Tucker Catlett and Holditch-Davis, 1990). However, swaddling may interfere with the functioning of radiant heaters and should be used with caution for infants with an unstable temperature and for babies nursed under a radiant warmer.

Non-nutritive sucking

Recommendations to use pacifiers to aid non-nutritive sucking for preterm infants have appeared in research-based nursing publications for a number of years, and should be a part of the gavage feeding procedure (Oehler, 1993). Non-nutritive sucking

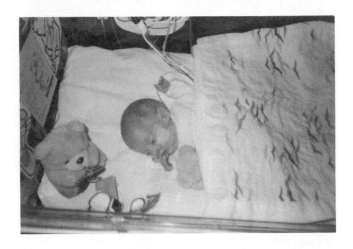

Figure 5.6 *An infant swaddled in a cot. The blanket is placed from the shoulders down, allowing hand-to-mouth behaviours, with the ends secured under the mattress.*

also decreases the behavioural and, to a lesser extent, physiological deterioration that often accompanies painful procedures (Field and Goldson, 1984; Tucker Catlett and Holditch-Davis, 1990) (Fig. 5.7). Thus, using a pacifier during unpleasant procedures and tube feedings may actually lessen some of the negative effects of environmental stress on the premature infant (Tucker Catlett and Holditch-Davis, 1990). The concern about possible association of pacifiers with painful procedures would seem unlikely unless the two events were paired very closely in time. To avoid this possibility, the pacifier should be given in advance of preparing the infant for the painful procedure (Oehler, 1993).

Sucking on a pacifier satisfies the infant's sucking needs and may facilitate early learning that satiety and sucking are

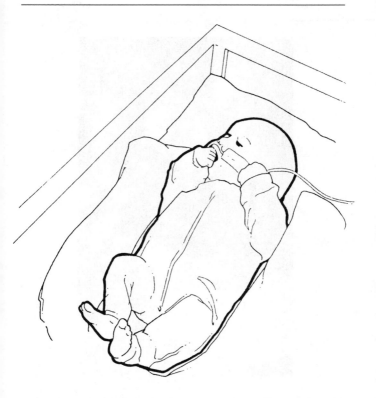

Figure 5.7 *Hand-to-mouth and non-nutritive sucking behaviours, reduce the behavioural and physiological deterioration that often accompany painful procedures.*

associated. However, nutritive and non-nutritive suckling are *not* alike. A baby who vigorously sucks on a pacifier may still not be able to suck nutritively, as the basis of nutritive suckling, the 'expressive' and 'swallow' phases, are not present in non-nutritive sucking (Merenstein and Gardner, 1993). This may be confusing for parents, requiring thorough explanation.

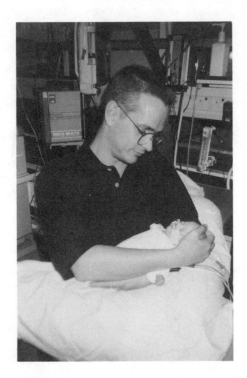

Figure 5.8 *Parents should be encouraged to hold, touch and rock their infant as the first tactile/kinesthetic stimulus for immature infants.*

Minimal handling protocol

Neonatal nurses are in a key position to act as advocates for preterm infants to protect them from unnecessary touch. However, the effectiveness of a minimal handling protocol, as outlined by the guidelines suggested, depends on the cooperation of all members of the multidisciplinary team.

Physiologically unstable infants may become overwhelmed

if simultaneously touched, talked to and visually aroused (Whitley and Cowan, 1991; Yecco, 1993). In these cases, it may be necessary to avoid talking to the infant or attempting to maintain eye contact during a procedure (Cole, 1985; Whitley and Cowan, 1991). Given the benefits of parents holding, touching and rocking their infants (Wolke, 1987), it would seem important to encourage these activities as the first tactile/kinesthetic stimuli for immature infants (Fig. 5.8). Further research is necessary to explore the effects of more typical maternal behaviours on weight gain and behaviour of preterm infants (Harrison and Woods, 1991; Oehler, 1993).

A review of the literature shows that, for preterm infants, handling must be based on two critical components: timing and individualization of care-giving. The key to appropriate intervention is generally the response of the care-giver to cues given by the infant. Recommendations for handling during care-giving and tactile/kinesthetic stimulation are included in the Protocol for Developmental Care of the Premature Infant (Appendix B).

CHAPTER SIX

Neuromotor Development

Effects of positioning on the preterm infant

INCREASING evidence suggests that supportive positioning and handling of premature infants may promote more normal motor development and minimize the chances of developing abnormal movement patterns (Bellefeuille-Reid and Jakubek, 1989; Bottos and Stefani, 1982; Fay, 1988; Jorgensen, 1993; Perez-Woods *et al.*, 1992; Turrill, 1992; Warren, 1993; Young, 1994).

The literature reviewed focused on four key areas when considering optimal positioning for the premature infant:

1 Prone *versus* supine positioning with effects on oxygenation and energy expenditure
2 Shoulder development
3 Cranial moulding
4 Hip posture

Only one study by Bozynski *et al.* (1988) addressed the effects of lateral positioning.

Prone versus *supine positioning*

In many neonatal units it was once accepted practice to nurse ill, premature infants supine, for ease of observation and to accommodate such equipment as umbilical artery catheters and ventilatory apparatus (Lioy and Maginello, 1988). However, several recent studies have suggested that supine positioning may not be optimal for the compromised infant in terms of oxygen and energy expenditure. Infants nursed in the prone position demonstrate increased oxygenation, tidal volume and lung compliance (Lioy and Maginello, 1988; Masterson *et al.*, 1987; Wagaman *et al.*, 1979, cited by Jorgensen, 1993; Warren, 1993), a reduction in the associated problems of apnoea of prematurity (Kurlak *et al.*, 1994), reduced energy expenditure (Masterson *et al.*, 1987), increased time asleep (Masterson *et al.*, 1987; Warren, 1993) and less activity, slower heart rate and more stable respiration (Brackbill *et al.*, 1973, cited by Fay, 1988) than when the same infants were placed supine. The prone position, together with the mattress elevated at 30°, is also associated with improved cardiovascular, pulmonary and gastrointestinal function (Perez-Woods *et al.*, 1992) (Fig. 6.1).

Nurses Fox and Molesky (1990) investigated the relationship between arterial oxygenation (P_aO_2) and supine–prone positions in preterm neonates with respiratory distress syndrome (see Table 2.3). Continuous arterial oxygen levels were measured during a 15-minute period for each infant ($n=25$) in both supine and prone positions. Results indicated a mean P_aO_2 of 71.5 mmHg for the prone position compared with 65.2 mmHg for the supine position, which is supported by previous studies (Lioy and Maginello, 1988; Wagaman *et al.*, 1979, cited by Jorgensen,

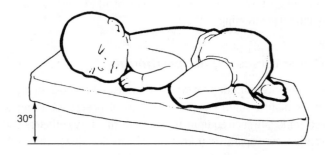

Figure 6.1 *The prone position, together with elevating the mattress 30°, is associated with improved cardiovascular, pulmonary and gastrointestinal function.*

1993). The researchers concluded that prone positioning results in improved oxygenation compared with supine positioning.

However, certain limitations of this study must be considered. The sample population was restricted to intubated premature infants with respiratory distress syndrome. Findings may not apply to term infants or those with other disease conditions, or in the absence of intubation or mechanical ventilation. The baffled water beds used placed less pressure on each infant's abdomen than may be achieved by different water beds or mattresses. Subjects were also studied in a deep sleep to minimize effects of behavioural state on P_aO_2. It is unknown whether differences in arterial oxygenation between the two positions would have been maintained if the subjects had been studied for longer than 15 minutes in each position. Despite these limitations, this study highlighted the importance for nurses to be aware of implications of positioning on respiratory functioning and to integrate this knowledge into their practice (Fox and Molesky, 1990).

Additional disadvantages of prolonged supine positioning

have been documented. These include increased startle responses and sleep disturbances (Fay, 1988; Whitley and Cowan, 1991) and an increased incidence of neck hyperextension and shoulder elevation in ventilated infants with respiratory distress syndrome (Anderson and Auster-Leibhaber, 1984, cited by Fay, 1988).

Shoulder development

Georgieff and Bernbaum (1986) also found that 46% of preterm infants studied demonstrated abnormal scapular retraction at 18 months of age. Scapular abduction and retraction limits the ability of the infant to rotate the shoulders forward, and thus sit without support, crawl, reach for objects, and manipulate or transfer objects, which are developmental tasks important in the first year of life (Bly, 1981, cited by Georgieff and Bernbaum, 1986). This 'arching' behaviour seen in so many chronically ill, premature infants may lead to difficulties in flexing the child when being nursed, cuddled, carried or dressed by parents and carers, which Pym (1992) postulated may have consequences for parental bonding.

Cranial moulding

Progressive head flattening, due to the weight of a large head resting laterally on the surface because of poor neck muscle tone, results in craniofacial deformation (Cubby, 1991). This is characterized in preterm infants by a 'high, narrow forehead with eyes that seem laterally placed in a long, narrow face' (Turrill, 1992, p. 25). The significance of a mis-shapen head is more than cosmetic. The normal rotation of an elliptical head in the supine position is difficult as the infant matures and neck muscle tone improves (Updike *et al.*, 1986).

Various aids thought to reduce bilateral head flattening have been investigated. These include water pillows (Marsden, 1980; Schwirian *et al.*, 1986, cited by Cubby, 1991), water beds (Hemingway and Oliver, 1991; Kramer and Pierpoint, 1989, cited by Cubby, 1991) and soft air-filled mattresses (Cartlidge and Rutter, 1988) (Fig. 6.2). Results were not conclusive and samples were small (Cubby, 1991; Young, 1994). No studies have evaluated the effectiveness of the soft, doughnut-shaped head supports reported to be used in many American neonatal units (Budreau, 1987; Cubby, 1991), and at present there are no controlled studies that indicate how positioning and regular turning of the head can be used to prevent craniofacial deformation. The frequency of head-turning practices in neonatal units is reported to vary significantly from 2 to 6 hours (Cubby, 1991), with some authors (Schwirian *et al.*, 1986, cited by Cubby, 1991) recommending that infants spend periods of time supported in the supine position to reduce cranial moulding.

Several papers have suggested that premature babies are

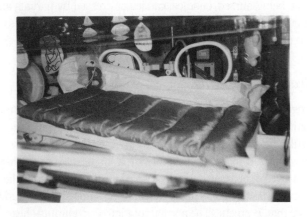

Figure 6.2 *Example of a soft 'Spenco' mattress used in many NICUs in the UK.*

often perceived by parents and care-givers as less attractive than their term counterparts (Alley, 1981; Budreau, 1987; Cubby, 1991; Hemingway and Oliver, 1991) and may even be at risk of increased child abuse and neglect (Elmer and Gregg, 1979; Maier *et al.*, cited by Cubby, 1991; Pym, 1992). However, one must use caution before generalizing these findings to parents of preterm babies, as attachment begins prenatally and other factors including the infant's behaviour and parental characteristics may influence the process.

Although much of the literature advocates prone over supine positioning for preterm babies, the prone position is not without problems. Delay in recognizing upper airway obstruction, abdominal distension and leakage of blood from umbilical artery catheters may occur if the infant is nursed prone. Left untreated, fatal sequelae may result (Munro, 1988).

Hip posture and supportive positioning

Downs *et al.* (1991), Turrill (1992) and Pym (1992) share the view that prolonged lying, supine *or* prone, may result in excessive hip flexion and flattened frog-like postures. Downs and colleagues (1991) investigated whether maintaining functional postures during hospital admission prevented the development of frog-lying or flattened postures in preterm infants who were randomly assigned to receive positioning according to usual nursing practice for the unit (control group, $n=24$) or specific hip support commencing at 7 days of age and continuing until the baby was at least a corrected age of 36 weeks (intervention group, $n=21$) (see Table 2.3).

Paediatricians assessed posture of the babies when gestational plus postnatal age of 40 weeks was reached, using standards formulated in a preliminary study based on the postural assessment of 25 full-term infants judged to be medically well.

The researchers concluded that specific hip support during the periods of intensive care results in fewer features of flattened posture at the age equivalent to term, with the effect significantly more noticeable in infants born at 24–28 weeks' gestation.

Although these results have implications directly applicable to nursing practice, and have already become influential in some clinical areas (Pym, 1992; Young, 1994), several limitations of this study must be considered. Although paediatricians performing the 40-week postural assessment at the follow-up clinic were unaware of the group to which each infant had been assigned, to minimize the risk of 'expectation' or 'diagnostic suspicion bias' (Page and Cusson, 1993), the method used to determine inter-observer reliability and the actual values calculated were not reported, restricting interpretation of the results (Holditch-Davis and Conway, 1993). Some infants were also discharged home before the postural assessment, however home environment and care, variables known to influence outcome (Page and Cusson, 1993), were not reported.

Despite these limitations, research in this area is to be welcomed as it appears to be one of the first quantitative assessments of supportive positioning, even though these techniques have been recommended since 1986 (Updike *et al.*, 1986). Follow-up studies, however, are essential to investigate whether these suggested practices will have deleterious effects on the long-term development of these infants. For, as Dunn (1991, p. 801) warned in a commentary of the research performed by Downs and colleagues, 'their conclusions as to what positions and postures are "normal" and "abnormal" must be treated with reservation…no weightbearing posture can be considered normal for the extremely premature infant'.

Recommendations for clinical practice

From a review of available literature it is evident that the primary aim of positioning management for the preterm infant is to encourage a balance between flexion and extension. Providing support to position the extremities toward the midline and to maintain body symmetry will promote a better balance of flexor and extensor musculature and prevent abnormal posturing and malformations, which in turn facilitates the development of normal movement patterns throughout infancy (Hallsworth, 1995; Whitley and Cowan, 1991). Downs *et al.* (1991), Pym (1992), Turrill (1992) and Young (1994) are advocates of supportive positioning in a variety of prone, lateral and supine positions to achieve this objective.

Frequent changes in position so that weight-bearing forces are not permitted to persist for prolonged periods in any one direction would be a fundamental principle on which guidelines for supportive positioning within the neonatal unit could be based (Young, 1994).

Prone positioning

There is consensus in the literature that prone positioning is preferred when physiological stability is the most important goal for the preterm infant (Fox and Molesky, 1990; Masterson *et al.*, 1987; Munro, 1988; Perez-Woods *et al.*, 1992; Warren, 1993; Young, 1994). Even the most acutely ill infant with assisted ventilation, umbilical artery catheters or chest tubes can be placed prone (Lawhon and Melzar, 1988; Whitley and Cowan, 1991) to facilitate lung excursion and improve oxygenation.

Prone positioning encourages flexion of all extremities and is best accomplished with a hip roll (Fig. 6.3) to prevent external rotation of the hip (Barb and Lemons, 1989; Downs *et al.*, 1991).

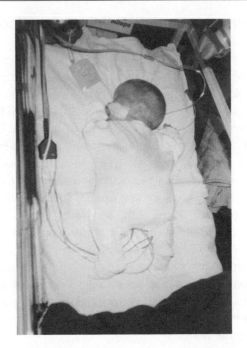

Figure 6.3 *Prone positioning: encourage flexion and adduction at hips and knees, and prevent external rotation of the hip, by placing a roll under the hips and possibly under the feet. Note hand-to-mouth behaviours encouraged in this position.*

The baby is positioned with some pelvic elevation so that the lower limbs are bearing weight through the anterior knee, and the hips are not flexed to more than 90° (Downs *et al.*, 1991; Hallsworth, 1995). Additional rolls or a 'nest' (Fig. 6.4) can be placed on either side of the infant to provide tactile stimulation and containment (Fay, 1988; Whitley and Cowan, 1991; Young, 1994). Babies who are contained tend to be calmer, to require less medication and to gain weight more rapidly

(a)

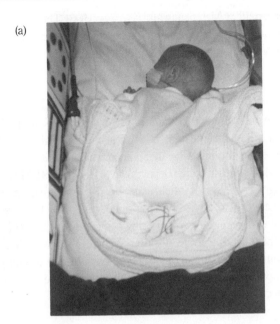

(b)

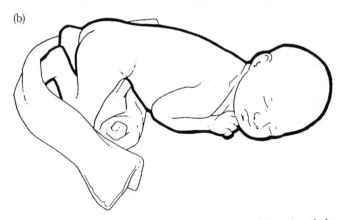

Figure 6.4 (a+b) *Rolls can be used to provide a 'nest' for containment and support of the infant placed prone.*

(Jorgensen, 1993; Merenstein and Gardner, 1993). The hands can also be brought close to the infant's mouth, promoting hand-to-mouth orientation and a calming effect (Fay, 1988; Jorgensen, 1993).

Sudden infant death syndrome

Research into sleeping position and the incidence of sudden infant death syndrome has shown that nursing babies in the prone position has an associated link, and should not be recommended for babies at home (Department of Health, 1991; Mitchell and Engelberts, 1991; Wigfield *et al.*, 1992). It is of great importance, therefore, to advise parents that, while their baby is in hospital with respiratory monitoring devices *in situ*, it is safe to nurse them in the prone position. Neonatal nurses need to accustom the infants to side or supine lying before discharge. Prone postioning thus appears to have both positive and negative effects when used for long periods.

Side-lying

If an infant cannot be placed prone, side-lying is preferable to the supine position (Bellefeuille-Reid and Jakubek, 1989; Turrill, 1992). In the lateral position, the trunk should be supported perpendicular to the cot surface (Downs *et al.*, 1991); this can be maintained by providing a wedge or rolled blanket behind the back with a folded sheet placed across the pelvis to maintain stability and flexion. A soft roll placed between the infant's legs will maintain neutral lower extremity positioning (Downs *et al.*, 1991; Hallsworth, 1995) (Fig. 6.5a). Pym (1992) also advocates placing a small nappy under the supporting hip to rotate the pelvis slightly and assist in flexion of the upper leg so that it may rotate and rest on the mattress (Fig. 6.5b). Moon-shaped rolls at the back or cut out foam have been used successfully in some units to facilitate appropriate side-lying (Whitley and Cowan, 1991) (Fig. 6.5c). To prevent arching against this back support, a soft roll or thin, stuffed toy can be provided to encourage the infant to flex toward the roll or toy (Fay, 1988) (Fig. 6.6). This position also allows flexion of the arms to facilitate sucking and self-calming behaviours (Turrill, 1992; Whitley and Cowan, 1991).

Supine positioning

If the baby must lie supine, support in a state of flexion is advocated (Fay, 1988; Turrill, 1992; Whitley and Cowan, 1991). The infant's knees and arms need to be lifted from the cot surface and supported, in order to reduce hip and shoulder abduction (Hallsworth, 1995) (Fig. 6.7). The head, body and feet can be supported in the midline, using soft blanket rolls positioned close to the baby (Turrill, 1992) to provide boundaries that contain the infant's movements and more closely approximating the womb (Fay, 1988; Vandenberg, 1985) (Fig. 6.8). An inverted 'halo' is also helpful in creating boundaries, and allows for head rotation (Hallsworth, 1995; Turrill, 1992). Special attention is needed when using padded rings as 'halos' as increased areas of pressure may result. It is advised that any 'halos' made to create boundaries around the infant's head should consist of soft malleable material such as a rolled sheet. A foam mattress with middle cut-outs to form a nest for the infant's trunk and head have also been used successfully in NICUs to maintain a supportive supine position (Hallsworth, 1995; Whitley and Cowan, 1991). Supporting the head in the midline position also minimizes the risk of apnoea, intermittent airway obstruction and fluctuations in intracranial pressure, which may result when the neck is turned to the side (Perez-Woods *et al.*, 1992). Small rolls can be placed under the knees to facilitate leg flexion, and

(a)

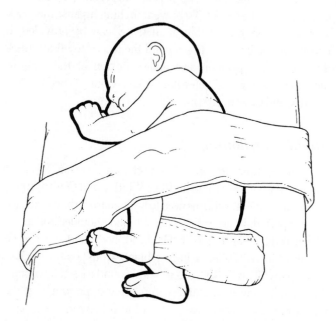

Figure 6.5 (a–c) *The lateral position can be maintained with a rolled blanket or wedge behind the back and through the legs, with a folded sheet placed across the pelvis.*

under the occiput if necessary to support the baby's airway, also allowing slight flexion of the head forward to minimize arching behaviour (Fay, 1988; Turrill, 1992).

Positioning aids

Supporting the feet by bracing them with a nest or rolls can help control movement, increase flexion and promote calming (Als, 1986; Cole, 1985). Often, babies are observed to have migrated

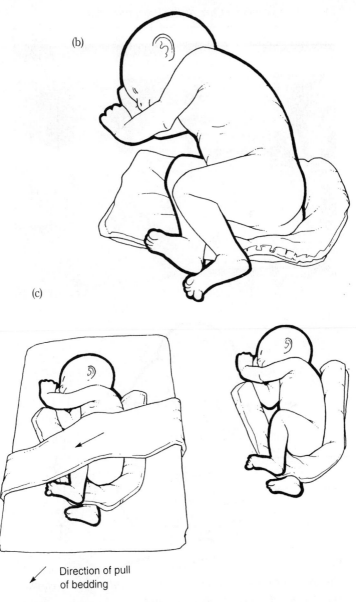

(b)

(c)

/ Direction of pull
of bedding

Figure 6.5 (a–c) *continued*

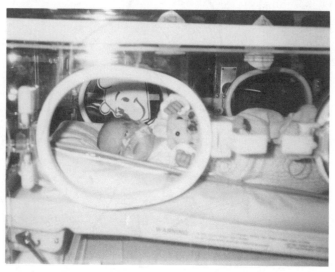

(a)

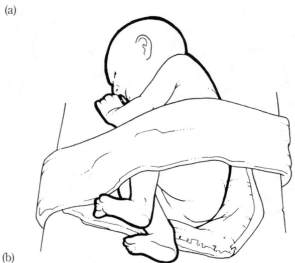

(b)

Figure 6.6 (a+b) *Sidelying: provision of a soft roll or toy encourages the infant to flex towards the object.*

Table 6.1 *Appropriate positioning: objectives and suggestions for support*

Position	Means of support	Reference
Prone		
Hands to face	Support from below arms	Hallsworth (1995)
Shoulders protracted	Soft moulding mattress	Whitley and Cowan (1991)
Spine curled	Soft mattress	Whitley and Cowan (1991)
Pelvic elevation (weight-bearing through anterior knee)	Padded roll under hips	Downs *et al.* (1991)
Knees bent and tucked in	Support for feet	Downs *et al.* (1991)
Feet at right angles	Support to push against	Downs *et al.* (1991)
Side-lying		
Head midline:	Soft mattress or small fluid-filled pillow	Cubby (1991)
Back slightly rounded	Moon shaped roll or foam	Whitley and Cowan (1991)
Stability and flexion	Support roll at spine	Downs *et al.* (1991)
Prevent arching	Soft stimulus to reach	Fay (1988)
Shoulders neutral or protracted (not retracted)	Roll in front to reach	Fay (1988)
	Shaped support at baby's back	Grunwald and Becker (1991)
Hands to face	Containment	Whitley and Cowan (1991)
Knees flexed	Roll for feet to push against	Turrill (1992)
Symmetry	Support between legs	Downs *et al.* (1991)
Supine		
Head midline	Soft moulding mattress and/or 'halo'	Hallsworth (1995)
Symmetry and containment	Lateral support through nests	Turrill (1992)
Arms forward and midline	Shoulder support	Hallsworth (1995)
Flexed hips and knees	Support under knees and/or at feet to brace against	Turrill (1992)

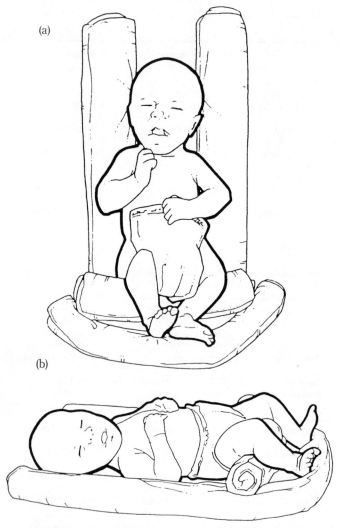

Figure 6.7 (a+b) *Supine: positioning small rolls lift and support the infant's arms and knees from the cot surface in order to reduce hip and shoulder abduction.*

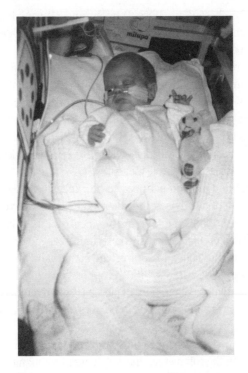

Figure 6.8 *"Nesting" or boundaries support an infant's position, assist energy conservation by containing movement and improve muscle tone by providing surfaces to flex against.*

to the periphery of the incubator to brace against its surface. By using 'nesting' and rolls, the baby will be supported (Table 6.1) and will not waste valuable calories migrating around the incubator. These supports also help to improve muscle tone as the baby has surfaces to flex against. The baby's security and stability may also be increased, so further reducing energy expenditure (Hallsworth, 1995; Merenstein and Gardner, 1993). Whenever possible, hands should be brought to the midline across the chest (Fay, 1988; Whitley and Cowan, 1991). Restraints should not be used to maintain a position (Oehler, 1993; Perez-Woods *et al.*, 1992; Whitley and Cowan, 1991).

Numerous interventions have been suggested as an attempt to prevent bilateral head flattening in preterm infants. These include water pillows, water beds, soft foam and air-filled mattresses, doughnut-shaped head supports and regular changes in head position to alternate sides (Cubby, 1991; Young, 1994). Further research is needed, however, to establish clearly the efficacy of these preventive measures.

Positioning aids do not need to be expensive. However, as Hallsworth (1995) advises, they do need to be attractive to look at, easy to store, and a suitable size for incubator use. Flannelette sheets in pastel colours or baby patterns are easy to launder and can be folded or rolled to appropriate shapes and sizes. These aids also provide parents with the opportunity to choose their infant's bedding, as the choice of clothes is often removed when the baby is very ill and needs to be nursed naked (Hallsworth, 1995).

In addition, positioning aids are becoming more readily available on the commercial market. Several companies in Britain, Europe and the USA have developed positioning supports suitable for use in special care baby units (SCBUs) and after discharge. Contact addresses are provided under Useful Addresses at the end of this book.

A team of research designers, led by rehabilitation designer Vivien Young, from 'Tools for Living' at the Brunel Institute for

Figure 6.9 (a–c) *The Positioning Bolster, available in several sizes (Prem Positioners; 'Tools for Living') can be used to assist the preterm infant to maintain supine, side-lying and prone positions. Adapted from Young, V. (1995) Tools for Living: Prem Positioners. Uxbridge: Brunel Institute for Bioengineering, Brunel University (with permission).*

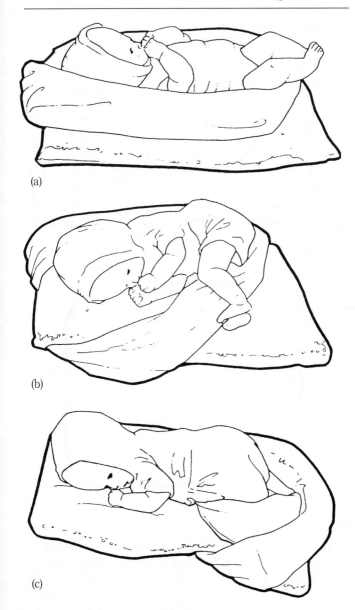

(a)

(b)

(c)

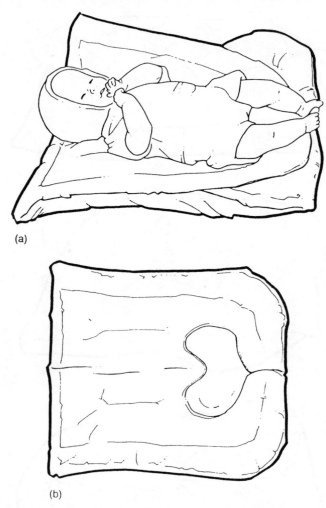

(a)

(b)

Figure 6.10 (a+b) *The Posture Mattress (Prem Positioners; 'Tools for Living'). In the supine position this aid supports the knees to create a more flexed posture and allows the hips to rotate forward. (c) Side-lying with Posture Mattress. Back support can be increased by*

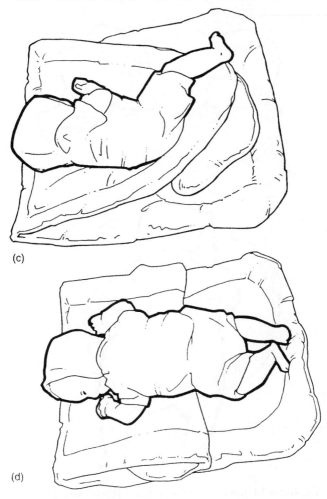

(c)

(d)

*means of additional padding beneath the mattress. (d) Prone posi-
tioning with the Posture Mattress supports the legs in a flexed
position. Adapted from Young, V. (1995) Tools for Living: Prem
Positioners. Uxbridge: Brunel Institute for Bioengineering, Brunel
University (with permission).*

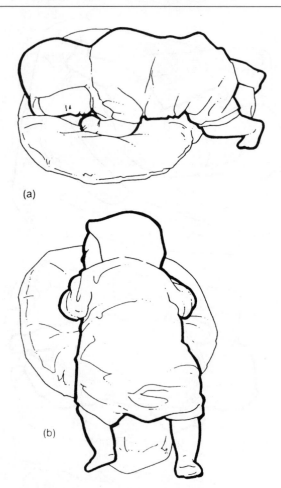

(a)

(b)

Figure 6.11 (a+b) *The Prone Pillow (Prem Positioners; 'Tools for Living'). Support under the hips reduces the flattened frog-like posture, allowing the legs to support the weight of the lower body. Adapted from Young, V. (1995) Tools for Living: Prem Positioners. Uxbridge: Brunel Institute for Bioengineering, Brunel University (with permission).*

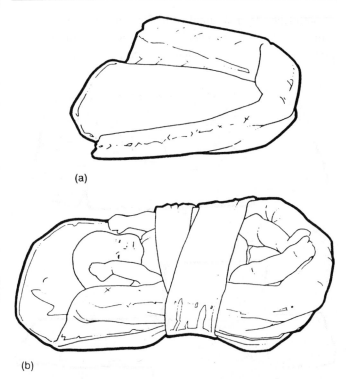

(a)

(b)

Figure 6.12 (a+b) *The Snug Nest (Prem Positioners; 'Tools for Living') provides comforting boundaries and enables the baby to be lifted safely with minimal disturbance. Adapted from Young, V. (1995) Tools for Living: Prem Positioners. Uxbridge: Brunel Institute for Bioengineering, Brunel University (with permission).*

Bioengineering, have developed a range of *Prem Positioners* for postural support of the preterm baby. These positioning supports, intended for commercial sale in the future, were developed in collaboration with a physiotherapist from University College Hospital, London, an occupational therapist from St Mary's Hospital in London, and nurses from the Special Care Baby Units at both Hillingdon Hospital and Wexham Park Hospital. The aim of the *Prem Positioners* is to encourage preterm babies to adopt flexed positions, similar to those that a full-term baby

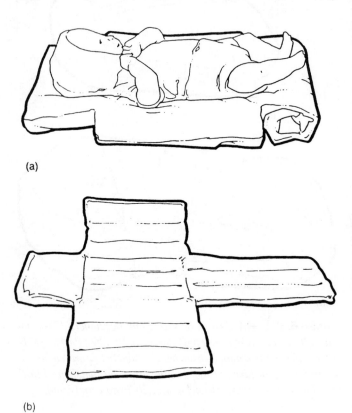

(a)

(b)

Figure 6.13 (a+b) *The Ribbed Mattress (Prem Positioners; 'Tools for Living') provides a soft mallable surface and allows the baby's position to be changed from a side-lying to a prone or supine position with minimal disturbance. Adapted from Young, V. (1995) Tools for Living: Prem Positioners. Uxbridge: Brunel Institute for Bioengineering, Brunel University (with permission).*

assumes naturally, with the objective to provide appropriate postural support for each individual baby's requirements. Examples of some *Prem Positioners* are featured in Figs 6.9–6.13. It is intended that this range of positioning supports will be developed further, and that an educational training package for SCBU nurses will be produced to promote the importance of positioning as part of the general nursing care of preterm babies (Young, 1995) (see Useful Addresses for contact address).

Conclusion

Evidently positioning of preterm infants is an area requiring further investigation (Cubby, 1991; Downs *et al.*, 1991; Young, 1994). In the meantime, neonatal nurses can utilize their key positions to implement suggested interventions and improve the long-term neuromotor development of these infants (Fay, 1988; Young, 1994). Recommendations for supportive positioning are included in the Protocol for Developmental Care of the Premature Infant (Appendix B).

CHAPTER SEVEN

Conclusion

WITH ADVANCED technologies and highly skilled nursing care, premature infants have a greater chance of survival. Accompanying this survival is the risk of visual, auditory, somatosensory and neurodevelopmental deficits (Shultz, 1992). The development of the infant is linked to the dynamic interaction of the infant with the environment (Als, 1986). There is consensus in the literature that the high-tech environment of the neonatal intensive care unit (NICU) is not appropriate for the immature developing central nervous system of the premature infant (Als, 1986; Avery and Glass, 1989; Becker *et al.*, 1991; Gardner Cole *et al.*, 1990; Oehler, 1993; Shultz, 1992; Vandenberg, 1985; White-Traut and Hutchens Pate, 1987). Thus neonatal practitioners must critically analyse and modify the NICU environment to support the development of preterm, medically fragile infants (Heriza and Sweeney, 1990).

Nursing interventions that provide developmental support facilitate behavioural organization through the promotion of self-regulating behaviour (Yecco, 1993). Infants who can maintain or regain physiological and behavioural organization will conserve energy for growth; provide care-givers with clear

behavioural cues that indicate their needs; facilitate the estab-
lishment of parent–infant attachment; and use self-consoling or
habituating behaviours when interacting with an environment
that is too stimulating (Als, 1986; Blanchard, 1991; D'Apolito,
1991). As a result, developmental outcome can be enhanced,
particularly in premature infants who are at risk of neurobehavioural sequelae and developmental delay (D'Apolito,
1991).

Empirical studies by Als *et al.* (1986) and Becker *et al.* (1991)
will be discussed to demonstrate how the integration of many
of the components of the developmental approach to care, reviewed in the preceding four chapters, has resulted in significant
improvements in outcome for premature infants.

Individualized nursing care

Avery and Glass (1989) proposed that a rational programme of
nurture in the NICU must begin with reference to each individual
premature infant, as sensory modalities do not all mature at the
same time. This proposal is supported by research which suggests that individualized nursing care based on behavioural
assessments of premature neonates can improve developmental
outcome for these infants (Als *et al.*, 1986; Becker *et al.*, 1991,
1993; D'Apolito, 1991; Jorgensen, 1993; Oehler, 1993; Peters,
1992; Shultz, 1992; Resnick *et al.*, 1987).

NIDCAP

The Neonatal Individualized Developmental Care and Assessment Programme (NIDCAP) is an approach proposed by Als
(1986) which requires care-givers to observe sensitively each
infant's behavioural response to each environmental event.

Table 7.1 *The nursing role in developmental intervention*

GOALS

1 Reduce stress experienced by the preterm infant
2 Increase self-regulatory behaviours of the preterm infant

METHOD

Assess	Observe behavioural cues displayed by the individual preterm infant to its environment. Assess environment and care for factors that may be potentially stressful for the preterm infant.
Plan	Collaborate with parents in formulating a developmental care plan based on research-based recommendations which will meet the individual infant's needs.
Implement	Integrate developmental interventions into daily nursing care of the preterm infant, in collaboration with the family and ancillary health professionals.
Evaluate	Determine the impact and effectiveness of the interventions meeting the individual preterm infant's needs, as demonstrated by the infant's behavioural responses to its environment.

Utilizing the synactive theoretical model proposed by Als (1986) and systematic NIDCAP observation of the infant's behaviours, an individualized care plan can be implemented. Based on the behaviours displayed by each infant, the immediate environment and the care-giving therapeutic approach are adapted to the infant's specific needs. The goals of these adaptations are to facilitate the reduction of stress behaviours and the increase of self-regulatory behaviours (Gardner Cole *et al.*, 1990). The approach is highly individualized and adapted to each infant's specific level of maturation (Als, 1986) (Table 7.1, Fig. 7.1).

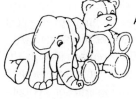

A DEVELOPMENTAL CARE PLAN FOR :

MY STRENGTHS ARE :

TIME OUT SIGNALS :

THESE THINGS STRESS ME :

HOW YOU CAN HELP ME :

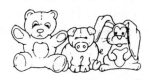

Figure 7.1 *Format for an individualized developmental care plan.*

Parental involvement

The NIDCAP approach advocates direct parental involvement in the planning of the services and needs of their infant (Als, 1986; Blanchard, 1991). Nurses can help parents to identify the degree of stimulation tolerated by their infant and the behavioural cues that invite or attempt to avoid interaction (Tribotti and Stein, 1992; Yecco, 1993). Culp and colleagues (1989) documented that parents who were given the opportunity to observe their infant's behavioural capabilities during the Assessment of Preterm Infant Behaviour—the NIDCAP assessment tool—had more realistic perceptions of their infant; that fathers had less anxiety; and that mothers seemed more aware of their premature infant's attempt to withdraw from disturbing stimulation.

Broadening the knowledge, skills and experience of parents by teaching them to recognize infant signals early has been documented to increase involvement in infant caretaking by improving parents' perceptions of their infant's abilities (Barb and Lemons, 1989; Cusson and Lee, 1994); to improve parenting skills (Als, 1986; Field, 1986; Yecco, 1993); and to enhance infant development (Field, 1986; Yecco, 1993). Parents who receive emotional support and information, and who participate in their infant's care, cope better with the crisis of premature birth (Cusson and Lee, 1994; Oehler, 1993). Thus parent participation in decision-making and actual hands-on experience in caring for their child in preparation for their role as full-time parents is recommended as essential (Cusson and Lee, 1994; Shultz, 1992; Oehler, 1993), and is proposed by Wright Lott (1989) as the key to successful developmental intervention.

Benefits of developmental care

An individualized developmental approach to care is now being widely advocated on the basis of studies that have demonstrated the positive effects of many of its components (Becker *et al.*, 1991; Shultz, 1992; Oehler, 1993; Whitley and Cowan, 1991; Wright Lott, 1989; Wolke, 1987). There are, however, few studies documenting the beneficial effects of such a programme as a whole (Becker *et al.*, 1991).

An initial study by Als *et al.* (1986) found that assessing the individual infant's ability to cope with excessive stimulation provided the care-giver with information to modify each infant's environment and treatment strategies. Significant outcome improvements were evidenced by fewer days on assisted ventilation; shorter time taken to progress from gavage feedings to breast or bottle feeds; shorter hospital stay by 2–6 weeks; a marked reduction in the number of complications; and improved neurodevelopmental outcome during the first 18 months of life. Results from two recent studies, a five-site multitrial study by Als *et al.* (1993, cited by Jorgensen, 1993) and a study by Vandenberg *et al.* (1993, cited by Jorgensen, 1993), have replicated the earlier work of Als and colleagues. In all these studies, each infant was cared for by a formally trained, primary care nurse who developed care plans based on periodic, systematic behavioural observation performed by expert clinicians. This level of expertise is not, however, available in most NICUs (Becker *et al.*, 1991).

Research findings by Becker *et al.* (1991) extend those of Als and colleagues (1986) by demonstrating that the beneficial effects of developmental care can be achieved with the resources available in most NICUs. Individualized developmental care was implemented by means of a general programme of nursing staff education and accompanied by ongoing support and consultation with the unit's neonatal clinician and occupational therapist to determine whether significant short-term outcomes, including medical and growth parameters during hospitalization and behavioural organization at discharge, could be achieved.

Guidelines for developmental nursing procedures were incorporated into standards of care for the unit following an education programme for staff nurses on the behaviour and development of the premature infant using the NIDCAP approach. The guidelines addressed five areas: (1) reduction in light and sound levels; (2) reduction of the stressful nature of medical and caretaking interventions by providing physical supports, promoting self-regulatory behaviours and allowing 'time-out' following periods of destabilization; (3) promoting sleep–wake organization by clustering care and reducing light levels during sleep; (4) promoting motor development by physical containment and flexed positioning and (5) providing opportunities for non-nutritive sucking during gavage feedings.

Experimental infants ($n=24$) demonstrated more optimal respiratory status, measured by oxygen saturation levels and the number of infants requiring oxygen at 28 days or more; reduced time taken to progress from gavage to oral feeding by an average of 6 days; lower levels of morbidity as assessed by the Neonatal Morbidity Scale measuring the incidence of 20 pathophysiological conditions; shorter hospitalization by an average of 2 weeks; and improved behavioural organization measured by the Neonatal Behavioural Assessment Scales, when compared with control infants ($n=21$). These results suggest that the developmental approach to nursing care of the preterm infant may have the potential to improve behavioural organization and reduce the continuing morbidity experienced by these infants (Becker *et al.*, 1991, 1993).

Controlled studies on the impact of developmental care protocols have been reported by Grunwald and Becker (1991) and by Jorgensen (1993) to have additional beneficial outcomes, including a decreased incidence of hypoxic episodes, intraventricular haemorrhage, bronchopulmonary dysplasia and retinopathy of prematurity; a reduction in the number of infants requiring long-term physical and occupational therapy; accelerated weight gain and improved parent–infant bonding.

These outcomes are important to consider in the light of current ethical and economic debates highlighted in recent media coverage relating to the setting of age–weight or gestational limits for care provided to preterm infants (Doyle, 1994). Increasingly parents, doctors and National Health Service managers are asking how far they should go in saving the lives of these tiny babies. In the UK the cost of neonatal care alone for premature babies weighing less than 3 lb is up to £70 million per year, with the cost of special education for resultant disabled children adding a further £150 million, according to calculations by the Office of Health Economics (Doyle, 1994).

Future research

Much research remains to be done. Developmental assessment tools that incorporate premature behaviour performance skills and predict developmental outcomes remain elusive (Dodd, 1994). From the research presented there is sufficient evidence to support reduced lighting and noise levels in the NICU setting and the consideration of cycled lighting periods. Safe levels of light in the NICU have not yet been established, and both timing and length of periods of darkness in relation to the 24-hour cycle and the infant's own sleep–wake cycles warrant additional investigation. Face-to-face visual stimulation would seem sufficient for infants less than 40 weeks old until further research has been carried out.

Further investigation of long-term effects of NICU noise on premature infants is indicated by the deficit in recent definitive documentation in this area (Lotas, 1992). Talking to infants who are in a state other than sleep is to be encouraged (Oehler, 1993), while planned interventions such as taped music and vocal selections require continued exploration.

There is a sufficient research base to support handling and caretaking that considers the state of the infant and aims to disrupt sleep as little as possible. Similarly, evidence for placing infants in ways to promote a balance of flexion and extension, and the prone position whenever possible, is well documented. However, further investigation into the effects of supportive positioning practices, e.g. specific hip support, on long-term development is advisable (Dunn, 1991). Interventions such as promotion of non-nutritive sucking and physical containment during feeding and handling are measures widely recommended to reduce stress responses in preterm infants (Oehler, 1993). Mantovani and Powers (1991) and Oehler (1993), however, warn that any stimulation intervention programme should be approached cautiously until the relative merits and possible adverse effects of the various interventions are known.

As nurses integrate these techniques into practice, nurse researchers and clinicians must design new studies to test the efficacy of specific interventions and determine the most effective interventions to support preterm infant development (Lawhon and Melzar, 1988; Dodd, 1994). Neonatal practitioners are challenged to continue the validation of NICU developmental intervention by participating in ongoing, risk–benefit, cost–benefit and efficacy studies (Dodd, 1994).

Role of the neonatal nurse

Developmental and behavioural assessment and intervention are concepts ideally suited to nursing which provides a model of holistic care (Treas, 1993). With nurses in the NICU providing more than 85% of care to critically ill infants (Peters, 1992), in intimate contact with their tiny patients, there is great potential for nursing intervention in the form of developmental care to optimize the long-term developmental outcomes for these vulnerable preterm babies.

Neonatal nurses are the key to the implementation of developmentally focused care for premature infants. By keeping informed of current developmental findings, implementing techniques to minimize detrimental stimuli and providing appropriate stimuli, the neonatal nurse can have a positive influence on the preterm infant's outcome. The most powerful influence on developmental outcome is the support and education of each infant's parents. The recommendations proposed in this book following critical analysis of current literature have been formulated into a Protocol for Developmental Care of the Premature Infant (Appendix B).

The guidelines presented form a resource foundation to assist neonatal nurses to develop creatively individualized plans of care for premature infants in collaboration with the family and ancillary health professionals. These interventions, when effectively implemented, have the potential to optimize the infant's early development and later functioning within society.

Relationships between Fetal Brain Development, Behavioural Organization and the Environment

INFANT DEVELOPMENT depends on the dynamic relationship between endowment and environment. Development is a continuous process from conception to maturation, and thus development of the infant is the beginning of the child, and ultimately of adult competence in the world. The relationship between endowment and environment is enhanced by review of the principles of development in Table A.1.

Table A.1 *Principles of development*

- Development is a continuous process from conception to maturation (i.e. development occurs *in utero* too).

- Growth and development are influenced by genetic make-up and environmental experiences.

- Development occurs in an orderly sequence, largely determined by readiness or maturation.

- The sequence of development is the same in all children; the rate of development is individual.

- Development is cephalocaudal (from head to foot) and from gross to specific (e.g. central to peripheral).

- The first 5 years of life are marked by a rapid period of growth of all body systems. During this time behaviour patterns are developed and are greatly influenced by the environment.

- Environmental stimulation provides conceptual development and influences level of intelligence.

- Learning occurs when behavioural change is not due solely to maturation; learning is facilitated by reinforcement of the behaviour.

- Development of the infant occurs within the framework of interaction with a caretaker and within the family.

Source: Merenstein and Gardner (1993, p. 565), with permission.

Development of the fetal brain

Premature infants are born as early as 16 weeks before usual term birth and their development is of concern because of the vulnerability of the developing central nervous system (Oehler, 1993). The developmental changes occurring in the brain between 24 and 40 weeks of gestation are considerable and correspond to the beginning of the most active period of organizational events (Blanchard, 1991). During this period the fetal brain should quadruple in size; cortical areas increase to the point of forming rich sulci and gyri; neuronal migration and organization, and the appearance of synaptic connections, are associated with greatly increased cortical activity and state control; and the fetus moves between differentiated sleep and wakefulness (Avery and Glass, 1989; Blanchard, 1991).

Full configuration of the brain takes place after birth and is guided by stimuli, information and challenges that originate in, and are specific to, a particular environment (Als, 1986; Blanchard, 1991). Thus the infant born prematurely is presented with the task of achieving homoeostasis in the presence of a large variety of stimuli-taxing systems that may not be ready for stimulation (Heriza and Sweeney, 1990). Additionally preterm babies are particularly vulnerable to intraventricular haemorrhage (IVH) associated with the tenuousness of the capillary bed and of vascular autoregulation, which is part of the normal brain development of the fetus at this stage (Als, 1986; Dietch, 1993; Kling, 1989). Moreover IVH is associated with hypoxic events (asphyxia, apnoea, hyaline membrane disease) leading to increased cerebral blood flow, impaired vascular autoregulation and increased venous pressure, which are all factors accompanying many of the events experienced by premature infants (Als, 1986).

Environmental influences

As developmental impairment is also present in infants spared the more massive insults of haemorrhage or hypoxaemic–anoxic events (Barb and Lemons, 1989), there is consensus in the literature (Als, 1986; Avery and Glass, 1989; Becker *et al.*, 1991; Oehler, 1993) that the environment influences the development of the preterm infant's brain through various senses: visual, auditory, cutaneous, tactile, somatesthetic, kinesthetic, olfactory and gustatory (Als, 1986).

Direct or indirect brain insults are a consequence of a mismatch between the extrauterine environment and the capacity of the central nervous system of the preterm infant, adapted for intrauterine existence, to adapt to the extrauterine environment (Als, 1986; Blanchard, 1991).

The neonatal intensive care unit (NICU) is clearly different from the intrauterine environment designed for the stages of central nervous system maturation. The intrauterine environment is warm and dark, with rhythmic background sounds and features physical containment with vestibular stimulation through the motions of the mother. By contrast the NICU is frequently bright, loud, intrusive, often painful and unrelenting. Cycles of rest and sleep are unintentionally, but repeatedly disrupted (Avery and Glass, 1989; Field, 1990; Langer, 1990).

In addition, premature infants rarely become large enough *in utero* to develop 'physiological flexion' and adopt the 'fetal position', believed essential to allow normal body movements and control to develop (Fay, 1988). Unable to nullify the force of gravity on skeletal tissues due to inadequate muscle tone, a premature infant is at risk of developing extended postures which may result in delays in normal motor development (Bly, 1981, cited by Fay, 1988) and postural and skeletal deformities (Young, 1994).

Researchers now propose (Blanchard, 1991; Gottfried and Gaiter, 1985; Heriza and Sweeney, 1990; Merenstein and Gardner, 1993) that rather than too much or too little stimulation, infants in the NICU receive an inappropriate *pattern* of stimulation. Thus stimuli should be controlled and matched as closely as possible to the needs and actual level of sensory integration capacities of the preterm infant (Als, 1986; Blanchard, 1991;

Heriza and Sweeney, 1990; Tribotti and Stein, 1992; Vandenberg, 1985; Yecco, 1993).

Behavioural development

Als (1986) has been influential in increasing contemporary understanding of neonatal behavioural development through the Synactive Model of Neonatal Behavioural Organization (Yecco, 1993). This theory describes the gradual unfolding of the infant's intra-organism subsystems: the autonomic system, which ensures the organism's baseline functioning; the motor system, with its recognizable flexor posture and limb and trunk movements; the state organizational system, with its distinct states of consciousness; and the attentional–interactive system with

Table A.2 *Subsystems of infant behaviour*

Subsystem	Behaviour
Autonomic (physiological functioning)	Respiration, heart rhythm, colour changes, visceral signals (bowel movements, gagging, hiccoughing)
Motor	Posture, muscle tone, movement
State organization	Range of states, movement between states, clarity of state
Attention or interaction (assessed during alert state)	Ability to alert, process and respond to stimulation from environment
Regulatory	Ability to integrate all subsystems and to return to state of balance and relaxation

Source: Barb and Lemons (1989, p. 11), adapted from Als (1986), with permission.

Table A.3 *Stress and defence behaviours*

Stress signal	Behaviour
Autonomic and visceral	Seizures; gagging, choking; spitting up; hiccoughing; gasping; coughing; sneezing; yawning; sighing; tremoring, startling; straining, as if producing a bowel movement; respiratory pauses, irregular respirations, breath-holding; colour changes to mottled, webbed, cyanotic or grey
Motor	Motor flaccidity or 'tuning out': trunkal, extremity or facial (gape face) flaccidity Motor hypertonicity: i) with hyperextension of legs (sitting on air, leg bracing), arms (airplaning, saluting) or trunk (opisthotonos) Finger splaying, facial grimacing, tongue extensions, high guard arm positions ii) With hyperflexion of trunk and extremities (fetal tuck, fisting) Frantic, diffuse activity; squirming Frequent twitching
State-related	Diffuse sleep or awake states with whimpering sounds, facial twitches and discharge smiling; eye floating, roving eye movements; strained fussing or crying, silent crying; staring; frequent active averting; panicked or worried alertness, hyperalertness; glassy-eyed strained alertness, lidded, drowsy alertness; rapid state oscillations, frequent building up to arousal; irritability and prolonged diffuse arousal; crying; frenzy and inconsolability; sleeplessness and restlessness

Source: Als (1986, p. 21), with permission.

Table A.4 *Self-regulatory and approach behaviours*

Autonomic stability	• Smooth respiration • Pink, stable colour • Stable viscera
Motoric stability	• Smooth, well modulated posture; • Well regulated tone • Synchronous, smooth movements with efficient motoric strategies (hand clasping, finger folding, hand-to-mouth manoeuvres, grasping, suck searching and sucking, hand holding and tucking)
State stability and attentional regulation	• Clear robust sleep states • Rhythmical robust crying • Effective self-quieting • Reliable consolability • Robust, focused, shiny-eyed alertness with intent and/or animated facial expression (frowning, cheek softening, mouth pursing to ooh-face, cooing, attentional smiling)

Source: Als (1986, p. 22), with permission.

its differentiated awake state that is capable of elaborated affective and cognitive receptivity and activity. A fifth subsystem, the self-regulatory subsystem, is found within each of the other four subsystems (Table A.2). These subsystems support and influence each other (hence the term synactive) in an environment appropriate for their development. The underlying theoretical formulation of the synactive theory is based on biphasic balancing between the approach to appropriate stimulation and the defence against, or avoidance of, inappropriate stimulation (Als, 1986). Infants display stress or approach behaviours in each of the subsystems (Tables A.3–A.5).

These behaviours are the methods by which babies commu-

Table A.5 *Five subsystems of intra-organism functioning in the neonate*

(1) AUTONOMIC
- Colour
- Tremor/startles
- Visceral
- Heart rate
- Respiratory rate

(2) MOTOR
- Tone
- Movement
- Activity
- Posture

(3) STATE
- Sleepy or drowsy
- Awake or alert
- Fussing or crying

(4) ATTENTION–INTERACTION
- Availability
- Alertness
- Robustness of interaction

(5) SELF-REGULATORY
- Autonomic or physiological
- Postural
- State changes

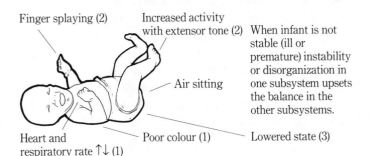

Good colour (1)   Even heart and respiratory rates (1)   Relaxed posture (2)

When infant is stable these subsystems work together, supporting and enhancing each other

Alert and active (4)   Awake and alert (3)
Hand to mouth (5)

Finger splaying (2)   Increased activity with extensor tone (2)   When infant is not stable (ill or premature) instability or disorganization in one subsystem upsets the balance in the other subsystems.

Air sitting

Heart and respiratory rate ↑↓ (1)   Poor colour (1)   Lowered state (3)

Adapted from Gardner Cole *et al.* (1990, p. 18), with permission.

Table A.6 *Behavioural responses of premature infants to their environment*

Cue	Behaviour
Disengagement (infant is overstimulated and needs to terminate the interaction)	Tongue thrusting, sagging cheeks, clenched fists, furrowed brow, hiccoughs, gaze aversion, splayed, extended fingers, yawning, frequent attempts to establish boundaries, arching of trunk or extremities, hyperalertness with a fearful expression on the face, air sitting (lower extremities extended out straight without support)
Subtle engagement (infant is able to initiate or continue an interaction)	Alerting, brow raising, assuming feeding posture (hands fisted, flexion of forearm, head raised, eyes directed upward to the care-giver)
Potent engagement	Sustained eye-to-eye contact, gazing directly at care-giver's face

Source: Barb and Lemons (1989, p. 9), with permission

nicate with care-givers to tell them what they need, how much and when (illustrated in Table A.6), and provide the avenue by which the brain and its functioning in the extrauterine environment may be assessed (Blanchard, 1991). Attention to preterm infants' individual behavioural cues, leading to appropriate changes in their environment and care, would result in a reduction of stress behaviours, an increase of specific self-regulatory behaviours and improved developmental outcome for these infants (Als, 1986; Als *et al.*, 1986; Becker *et al.*, 1991; Grunwald and Becker, 1991).

Protocol for Developmental Care of the Premature Infant

Recommendations for controlling environmental light in the special care baby unit

1 Maintain 60 foot-candle (ft-c) lighting in the SCBU for adequate visualization of infants (American Academy of Pediatrics, 1992).

2 Utilize dimmer switches on lights to reduce ambient room light throughout day and night (Glass, 1993).

(a) Reduce light levels at night to promote development of diurnal cycles (Blackburn and Patteson, 1991).

(b) Adjust light levels during day periods to foster state transition and periods of alertness or sleep, following assessment of the infant's behaviour (Blackburn and Patteson, 1991).

3 Turn off lights that are not in use (Lotas, 1992).

4 Utilize individual spot lights if necessary for procedures or closer observation, with 100 ft-c recommended for procedures (American Academy of Pediatrics, 1992).

5 Avoid occluding infant's eyes beyond what is necessary for phototherapy (Glass, 1993).

6 Utilize curtains or window shades to reduce direct sunlight exposure (Lotas, 1992).

7 Employ the use of screens to shield infants in incubators adjacent to those in which phototherapy is being used (Lotas, 1992).

8 Utilize dimmer switches to increase light intensity gradually following night cycles or procedures requiring near darkness, e.g. electrocardiography or ultrasonography, to reduce potential stress to infant caused by a sudden change in environmental illumination (Blackburn and Patteson, 1991).

9 *For preterm infants in a stable condition:*
Employ drapes partially to cover the incubator, crib or headbox, while ensuring visibility of the colour of fingers, toes and trunk, of positioning, and of equipment attached to baby. The nurse should use her clinical judgement of the baby's condition and the situation to determine whether an intervention should be employed at a particular time (Yecco, 1993).

10 Remove drapes when the infant's parents are visiting (Lotas, 1992).

11 *For preterm infants in an acutely ill condition:*
Ensure an unobstructed view of the critically ill infant while ambient light levels are reduced throughout the day and night (Treas, 1993).

Recommendations for controlling environmental noise in the special care baby unit

1 Conduct conversations and unit rounds away from incubators or outside the care-giving area if possible. Reduce talking to a whisper by the cotside (Strauch *et al.*, 1993).

2 Exclude radio use and intercom systems from the SCBU (Lotas, 1992).

3 Forward all phone calls to main office, separate from care-giving area (Strauch *et al.*, 1993).

4 Remove extraneous equipment, e.g. printers and centrifuges, from immediate care-giving area (Letko, 1992).

5 Minimize manipulation of large equipment in the care-giving area (Strauch *et al.*, 1993).

6 Consider machine noise when purchasing equipment (Letko, 1992).

7 Open and close incubator ports, doors, drawers and disposal bins with care (Yecco, 1993).

8 Respond rapidly to alarms or crying infants (Strauch *et al.*, 1993).

9 Set monitor alarms as low as practical (Letko, 1992).

10 Utilize drapes partially to cover the incubator, providing a padded interface to reduce environmental noise for stable infants (Treas, 1993).

11 Ensure water is removed frequently from ventilator tubing (Whitley and Cowan, 1991).

12 Find alternative methods to stimulate distressed infants, i.e. do not rap on incubator (Letko, 1992).

13 Utilize 'Quiet' signs to raise staff and parent awareness of the need to control environmental noise (Vandenberg, 1985).

14 Establish an intervention period of overall noise reduction in the SCBU (Strauch *et al.*, 1993).
15 Monitor noise levels inside unit incubators periodically to ensure limit of 60 decibels set by British Safety Standards is not exceeded (Horsley, 1990).

Recommendations for handling and touch during care-giving and social interaction in the special care baby unit

1 Identify individual stress signals and behavioural cues, and utilize these in organizing the infant's care according to individual tolerance levels (Cooper Evans, 1991).
2 Consolidate care during 'touch times': coordinate interactions and cluster activities while considering the infant's tolerance levels, to minimize handling and provide periods of uninterrupted rest (Jorgensen, 1993).
3 Evaluate whether the procedure is necessary or justifies the risk of alterations in oxygenation and sleep–wake states (Speidel, 1978).
4 Limit handling to essential procedures, particularly for critically ill infants requiring considerable support (Whitley and Cowan, 1991).
5 Ensure no procedure is allowed to continue for more than 15 minutes without a period of rest provided for the infant (Langer, 1990).
6 Assess infant's ability to tolerate each procedure before its commencement (Peters, 1992).
7 Suspend activity should the infant or monitor indicate a stress response to allow for recovery and to prevent severe or multiple hypoxaemic episodes (Cooper Evans, 1991).

8 Remain at the infant's cotside for at least 2–5 minutes following completion of any procedure (Peters, 1992).

9 Give infants with limited energy reserves more time to recover between care-giving activities or space out care over a longer time frame (Cooper Evans, 1991).

10 Ensure all supplies necessary to provide the infant's care are gathered before disturbing the infant (Lawhon and Melzar, 1988).

11 Coordinate blood sampling for laboratory tests and Dextrostix to be obtained with blood gas analysis via umbilical or venous catheters, to minimize the number of heel stabs (Whitley and Cowan, 1991).

12 Ensure invasive procedures, e.g. intravenous catheter insertions, lumbar punctures etc., are performed by the most skilled operator in the shortest possible time. If unsuccessful on the second attempt, allow the infant to recover before a further attempt is made (Speidel, 1978).

13 Utilize electronic monitoring apparatus to provide a continuous display and routine assessment of physiological parameters: respiratory and heart rates, blood pressure and temperature. Check parameters by auscultation and 'hands on' assessment once per shift to minimize handling (Langer, 1990).

14 Ensure suctioning is done according to need as assessed by breath sounds and respiratory status, never routinely (Langer, 1990).

15 Perform nappy changes in prone or side-lying position to minimize need for repositioning (Lawhon and Melzar, 1988).

16 Time care-giving activities to coincide with the infant's awake and more alert periods if possible (Whitley and Cowan, 1991).

17 Utilize alerting techniques, e.g. softly pitched voice, to rouse infant gently before care-giving procedure to prevent

startling, if disturbance during sleep is necessary (Whitley and Cowan, 1991).

18 Utilize special support strategies during procedures and interventions to promote self-regulatory behaviours, calm the infant, reduce agitation and minimize hypoxia:

(a) contain infant's extremities in flexed position with hands or swaddling;

(b) offer opportunities for grasping, using finger, cloth or pacifier handle;

(c) provide rest periods, 'time-outs', when infant shows marked signs of stress;

(d) maintain support following any aversive procedure or intervention until infant is calmed;

(e) offer pacifier and hold it in position (Grunwald and Becker, 1991).

19 Document and communicate techniques that are effective in the care of the infant as part of the neonate's individualized plan of care (Langer, 1990).

20 Implement individualized care based on the infant's responses to stimulation and duration of care-giving procedures (Cooper Evans, 1991).

21 Set aside specific 'hands off' rest periods during which all non-emergency procedures are postponed to assure infants an opportunity for undisturbed sleep and rest (Langer, 1990). Ensure awareness and cooperation with this protocol by multidisciplinary team members.

22 Utilize signs by the cotside to raise staff, parent and visitor awareness of minimal handling policies and the premature infant's need for rest.

23 Encourage parent participation with 'hands on' care, corresponding with infant 'touch times', closely monitoring for signs of intolerance during periods of stimulation (Langer, 1990).

24 Educate and guide parents to provide them with a better understanding of stress responses and to allow them to intervene in ways that conserve their infant's energy and structural and personal integrity (Langer, 1990).

25 Introduce massage and stroking stimuli cautiously, according to the infant's behavioural cues and tolerance levels. Encourage parental holding, touching and rocking as the first tactile or kinesthetic stimuli the infant receives (Oehler, 1993).

26 Ensure social interaction is initiated only during spontaneous quiet, alert states when the preterm infant is most resistant to stress (Tucker Catlett and Holditch-Davis, 1990).

Recommendations for supportive positioning in the special care baby unit

Aims of supportive positioning

- To stimulate active flexion of the trunk and limbs.
- To achieve more rounded heads and active head rotation.
- To encourage balance between extension and flexion.
- To allow for more symmetrical postures.
- To enhance midline orientation, which contributes to eye, hand and mouth control (Updike *et al.*, 1986).

Interventions

1 Utilize prone and side-lying positioning whenever possible. Utilize supine positioning only when prone or side-lying is not possible (Whitley and Cowan, 1991).

2 When positioning the infant prone:
(a) Keep the head in neutral position, or with the chin tucked

slightly toward the chest, to avoid hyperextension of the neck.

(b) Avoid total hip abduction (frog-leg position). Utilize soft roll under hips to support pelvis.

(c) Allow the hands to be in close proximity to the face (Grunwald and Becker, 1991).

3 When positioning the infant side-lying:

(a) Provide support so that the back is slightly rounded.

(b) Encourage hip and knee flexion.

(c) Keep the head in midline.

(d) Keep the upper shoulder in a neutral position (not re-tracted) (Grunwald and Becker, 1991).

4 When the infant must be placed in the supine position:

(a) Keep the head in midline or as close to the midline as possible.

(b) Encourage hip and knee flexion.

(c) Provide a support for foot bracing.

(d) Provide support behind the shoulder to help keep them slightly forward (Grunwald and Becker, 1991).

5 Utilize aids to achieve optimal positioning such as nests, blanket and nappy rolls, and sheepskins (Turrill, 1992).

6 Ensure that an infant's position is alternated on a regular basis, i.e. 4, 6 or 8-hourly, depending on the infant's condition (Grunwald and Becker, 1991). Document position on the nursing flowsheet, e.g. supine with head to right, left or midline (S@R, S@L or S@M); prone with head to right or left (P@R, P@L); or side-lying to right or left (SL@R, SL@L).

7 When lifting out of the incubator or repositioning, facilitate flexion and containment of extremities by using prone or lateral positions, or swaddling the infant (Whitley and Cowan, 1991).

8 Maintain mattress at 30° angle to promote cardiovascular,

pulmonary and gastrointestinal function (Perez-Woods *et al.*, 1992).

9   Enhance successful oral feeding behaviours with a semi-reclined, semi-flexed position with midline orientation. Sucking is part of the total flexor pattern and may be enhanced by giving the baby something to grasp (Warren, 1993).

10 Avoid unnecessary manipulation and repositioning of physiologically unstable infants (Whitley and Cowan, 1991).

Glossary

Decibel
Unit used to express the ratio of two powers, usually electrical or acoustic powers, equal to one-tenth of a bel; one decibel equals approximately the smallest difference in acoustic power the human ear can detect. Abbreviated dB (Miller and Keane, 1983).

Foot-candle
Unit of illumination being 1 lumen per square foot or equivalent to 1.0764 milliphots; cf. lux. Abbreviated ft-c (Albert, 1994).

Kinesthesia
The sense by which position, weight and movement are perceived. Adjective: kinesthetic (Miller and Keane, 1983).

Neurodevelopment
Defined as 'the early development of neonatal neurological systems in relation to normal development patterns' (Shultz, 1992, p. 11). Neurodevelopment relates to neurological status as assessed by observation of development and is the accepted shortened form of the term 'neurological development' (Barb and

Lemons, 1989). Neurological development of the newborn includes evaluation of (1) newborn reflexes, (2) neonatal states, (3) psychosocial interaction and (4) sensory capabilities. The neonate is born with behaviours that are unlearned, instinctual and of an adaptive and survival nature. They reflect the state of the nervous system and the level of neonatal maturation (Merenstein and Gardner, 1993).

Organization
In terms of infant development, the principles of organization involve establishing integrated functioning between the infant's physiological and behavioural systems (D'Apolito, 1991). The physiological system includes (1) autonomic functions that control the infant's heart rate, respiratory rate, oxygen saturation level, temperature, fluid balances, and enzyme and hormone production, and (2) visceral functions such as digestion and elimination. The infant's behavioural system is composed of motor activities and states of consciousness. The ability of these two systems to work in harmony is important for the infant's ongoing survival (Als, 1986; D'Apolito, 1991). An infant's physiological and behavioural systems function harmoniously to allow the infant to interact with the environment in an organized way. The organized infant is able to process external events without disrupting this physiological and behavioural functioning (Als, 1986; D'Apolito, 1991).

Preterm infant
Defined by the World Health Organization as an infant born at less than 37 completed weeks of gestation (less than 259 days) (Tudehope and Thearle, 1989).

Somatosensory system
Somatosensitivity (or somataesthesia) is consciousness or

awareness of, or sensibility to, bodily sensations (Gr *soma* body) (Miller and Keane, 1983).

Terminology

The terms neonatal intensive care unit (NICU), intensive care nursery and special care baby unit (SCBU) are used interchangeably throughout this book.

Transcutaneous oxygen tension

Trancutaneous oxygen tension ($P_{tc}O_2$) is a measurement of oxygen delivery from the respiratory system via the blood supply and into the tissue. Transcutaneous monitoring assists care-givers in the neonatal intensive care unit to keep an infant's arterial oxygen tension (P_aO_2) within safe limits. The $P_{tc}O_2$ will reveal any impairment of the infant's ability to deliver oxygen to the tissue and, because the skin ranks low in the body's system of oxygenation priority, provides the earliest possible warning of the onset of problems. Episodes of hypoxia, which may cause brain damage, and hyperoxia, which may cause retrolental fibroplasia, are quickly detected and thereby avoided (Baumbach, 1986).

References

Adamson, S. (1993) Hands-on therapy. *Health Visitor* **66**(2): 48–50.

Adamson-Macedo, E.N. (1986) Effects of tactile stimulation on low and very-low-birth-weight infants during the first year of life. *Current Psychological Research and Reviews* **Winter 1985–1986**: 305–306.

Adamson-Macedo, E.N. (1990) The effects of touch on preterm and fullterm neonates and young children. *Journal of Reproductive and Infant Psychology* **8**: 267–273.

Albert, D.M. (1994) Chief lexicographer, 'foot-candle'. In *Dorland's Illustrated Medical Dictionary*, 28th edn. Philadelphia, Pennsylvania: W.B. Saunders.

Alley, T. (1981) Head shape and the perception of cuteness. *Developmental Psychology* **17**(5): 650–654.

Als, H. (1986) A synactive model of neonatal behavioural organization: framework for the assessment of neurobehavioural development in the premature infant and for support of infants and parents in the neonatal intensive care environment. In Sweeney, J.K. (ed.) *The High-Risk Neonate: Developmental Therapy Perspectives*, pp. 3–53. New York: Haworth Press.

Als, H., Lawhon, G., Brown, E., Gibes, R., Duffy, F.H., McAnulty, G. and Blickman, J. (1986) Individualized behavioural and environmental care for the very low birth weight infant at risk for bronchopulmonary dysplasia: neonatal intensive care unit and developmental outcome. *Pediatrics* **78**(2): 1123–1132.

American Academy of Pediatrics (1992) *Guidelines for Perinatal Care*, 3rd edn. Elk Grove Village, Illinois: American Academy of Pediatrics.

Avery, G.B. and Glass, P. (1989) The gentle nursery: developmental intervention in the NICU. *Journal of Perinatology* **9**(2): 204–206.

Barb, S.A. and Lemons, P.K. (1989) The premature infant: towards improving neurodevelopmental outcome. *Neonatal Network* **7**(6): 7–15.

Barnes, C.A. and Kirchhoff, K.T. (1986) Minimising hypoxaemia due to endotracheal suctioning: a review of the literature. *Heart and Lung: The Journal of Critical Care* **15**(2): 164–177.

Barnett, K. (1972) A theoretical construct of the concepts of touch as they relate to nursing. *Nursing Research* **21**(2): 102–110.

Baumbach, P. (1986) *Understanding Transcutaneous pO_2 and pCO_2 Measurements*. Copenhagen: Radiometer.

Becker, P.T., Grunwald, P.C., Moorman, J. and Stuhr, S. (1991) Outcomes of developmentally supportive nursing care for very low birth weight infants. *Nursing Research* **40**(3): 150–155.

Becker, P.T., Grunwald, P.C., Moorman, J. and Stuhr, S. (1993) Effects of developmental care on behavioural organization in very-low-birth-weight infants. *Nursing Research* **42**(4): 214–220.

Bellefeuille-Reid, D. and Jakubek, S. (1989) Adaptive positioning intervention for premature infants: issues for paediatric occupational therapy practice. *British Journal of Occupational Therapy* **52**(3): 93–96.

Bernbaum, J.C., Pereira, G.R., Watkins, J.B. and Peckham, G.J. (1983) Non-nutritive sucking during gavage feeding enhances growth and maturation in preterm infants. *Pediatrics* **71**(1): 41–45.

Blackburn, S. and Patteson, D. (1991) Effects of cycled light on activity state and cardiorespiratory function in preterm infants. *Journal of Perinatal – Neonatal Nursing* **4**(4): 47–54.

Blanchard, Y. (1991) Early intervention and stimulation of the hospitalized preterm infant. *Infants and Young Children* **4**(2): 76–84.

Blanchard, Y., Pedneault, M. and Doray, B. (1991) Effects of tactile stimulation on physical growth and hypoxaemia in preterm infants. *Physical and Occupational Therapy in Pediatrics* **11**(1): 37–52.

Bodolf Rausch, P. (1981) Effects of tactile and kinesthetic stimulation on premature infants. *Journal of Obstetric, Gynecologic, and Neonatal Nursing* **10**(1): 34–37.

Booth, C.L., Johnson-Crowley, N. and Barnard, K.E. (1985) Infant massage and exercise: worth the effort? *MCN; American Journal of Maternal Child Nursing* **10**: 184–189.

Bottos, M. and Stefani, D. (1982) Postural and motor care of the premature baby. *Developmental Medicine and Child Neurology* **24**: 706–707.

Bozynski, M.E..A., Naglie, R.A., Nicks, J.J., Burpee, B. and Johnson, R.V. (1988) Lateral positioning of the stable ventilated very-low-birth-weight infant. *American Journal of Diseases of Children* **142**: 200–202.

Budreau, G. (1987) Postnatal cranial moulding and infant attractiveness: implications for nursing. *Neonatal Network* **5**(4): 13–19.

Burns, N. and Grove, S.K. (1993) *The Practice of Nursing Research: Conduct, Critique and Utilization*, 2nd edn, Philadelphia, Pennsylvania: W.B. Saunders.

Campbell, S.K. (1986) Organizational and educational considerations in creating an environment to promote optimal development of high-risk neonates. *Physical and Occupational Therapy in Pediatrics* **6**: 191–204.

Carruthers, A. (1992) A force to promote bonding and wellbeing: therapeutic touch and massage. *Professional Nurse* **February 1992**: 297–300.

Cartlidge, P.H.T. and Rutter, N. (1988) Reduction of head flattening in preterm infants. *Archives of Disease in Childhood* **63**(7): 755–757.

Clarke, R. (1992) Massage for babies. *International Journal of Alternative and Complementary Medicine* **10**(7): 13.

Cole, J.G. (1985) Infant stimulation re-examined: an environmental and behavioural based approach. *Neonatal Network* **3**(5): 24–31.

Compos, R.G. (1989) Soothing pain-elicited distress in infants with swaddling and pacifiers. *Child Development* **60**(4): 781–792.

Cooper Evans, J. (1991) Incidence of hypoxaemia associated with caregiving in premature infants. *Neonatal Network* **10**(2): 17–24.

Cubby, C. (1991) Craniofacial deformation in premature infants. *Paediatric Nursing* **3**(2): 19–21.

Culp, R.E., Culp, A.M. and Harmon, R.J. (1989) A tool for educating parents about their premature infants. *Birth* **16**(1): 23–26.

Cusson, R.M. and Lee, A.L. (1994) Parental interventions and the development of the preterm infant. *Journal of Obstetric, Gynecologic, and Neonatal Nursing* **23**(1): 60–68.

Danford, D.A., Miske, S., Headley, J. and Nelson, R.M. (1983) Effects of routine care procedures on transcutaneous oxygen in neonates: a quantitative approach. *Archives of Disease in Childhood* **58**: 20–23.

D'Apolito, K. (1991) What is an organized infant? *Neonatal Network* **10**(1): 23–29.

De Curtis, M., McIntosh, N., Ventura, V. and Brooke, O. (1986)

Effect of non-nutritive sucking on nutrient retention in pre-term infants. *Journal of Pediatrics* **109**(5): 888–890.

Degen Horowitz, F. (1990) Targeting infant stimulation efforts: theoretical challenges for research and intervention. *Clinics in Perinatology* **17**(1): 185–195.

Department of Health (1991) *Sleeping Position and the Incidence of Cot Death*. London: HMSO

Dietch, J.S. (1993) Periventricular–intraventricular haemorrhage in the very low birth weight infant. *Neonatal Network* **12**(1): 7–16.

Di Pietro, J.A., Cusson, R.M., O'Brien Caughy, M. and Fox, N.A. (1994) Behavioural and physiologic effects of non-nutritive sucking during gavage feeding in preterm infants. *Pediatric Research* **36**(2): 207–214.

Dodd, V. (1994) The evolution of neonatal developmental care: a personal journey. *Neonatal Network* **13**(6): 23–26.

Downs, J.A., Edwards, A.A., McCormick, D.C. and Stewart, A.L. (1991) Effect of intervention on development of hip posture in very preterm babies. *Archives of Disease in Childhood* **66**: 797–801.

Doyle, C. (1994) Tiny babies, huge decision. *Daily Telegraph* 19 July 1994.

Dunn, P.M. (1991) Commentary: Postural deformation of the newborn. *Archives of Disease in Childhood* **66**: 801.

Dyke, R.M. and Conway, A. (1992) Sampling neonatal popula-tions. *Neonatal Network* **11**(5): 75–77.

Ellison, P.H. (1984) Neurologic development of the high-risk infant. *Clinics of Perinatology* **11**(1): 41–58.

Elmer, E. and Gregg, G. (1979) Developmental characteristics of abused children. *Pediatrics* **40**: 596–602.

Ernst, J.A., Rickard, K.A., Neal, P.R., Yu, P., Oei, T.O. and Lemons, J.A. (1989) Lack of improved growth outcome related to non-nutritive sucking in very low birth weight premature infants fed a controlled nutrient intake: a randomized prospective study. *Pediatrics* **83**: 706–717.

Fanconi, S. and Duc, G. (1987) Intratracheal suctioning in sick preterm infants: prevention of intracranial hypertension and cerebral hypoperfusion by muscle paralysis. *Pediatrics* **79**(4): 538–543.

Fay, M.J. (1988) The positive effects of positioning. *Neonatal Network* **6**(5): 23–29.

Field, T. (1986) Interventions for premature infants. *Journal of Pediatrics* **109**: 183–191.

Field, T. (1990) Alleviating stress in newborn infants in the intensive care unit. *Clinics in Perinatology* **17**(1): 1–9.

Field, T. and Goldson, E. (1984) Pacifying effect of non-nutritive sucking on term and preterm neonates during heelstick procedures. *Pediatrics* **74**(6): 1012–1015.

Field, T.M., Schanberg, S.M., Scafidi, F. *et al.* (1986) Tactile/kinesthetic stimulation effects on preterm neonates. *Pediatrics* **77**(5): 654–658.

Field, T.M., Scafidi, F. and Schanberg, S. (1987) Massage of preterm newborns to improve growth and development. *Pediatric Nursing* **13**(6): 385–387.

Fox, M.D. and Molesky, M.G. (1990) The effects of prone and supine positioning on arterial oxygen pressure. *Neonatal Network* **8**(4): 25–29.

Gardner, S.L. and Hagedorn, M.I. (1990) Physiologic sequelae of prematurity: the nurse practitioner's role. Part II. Retinopathy of prematurity. *Journal of Pediatric Health Care* **4**(2): 72–76.

Gardner Cole, J.G., Begish-Duddy, A., Judas, M.L. and Jorgensen, K.M. (1990) Changing the NICU environment: the Boston City Hospital model. *Neonatal Network* **9**(2): 15–23.

Georgieff, M.K. and Bernbaum, J.C. (1986) Abnormal shoulder girdle muscle tone in premature infants during their first 18 months of life. *Pediatrics* **77**(5): 664–669.

Glass, P. (1993) Development of visual function in preterm infants: implications for early intervention. *Infants and Young Children* **6**(1): 11–20.

Glass, P., Avery, G.B., Subramanian, K.N.S., Keys, M.P., Sostek, A.M. and Friendly, D.S. (1985) Effect of bright light in the hospital nursery on the incidence of retinopathy of prematurity. *New England Journal of Medicine* **313**(7): 401–404.

Gordon Shogan, M. and Schumann, L.L. (1993) The effect of environmental lighting on the oxygen saturation of preterm infants in the NICU. *Neonatal Network* **12**(5): 7–13.

Gorski, P.A. (1985) Behavioural and environmental care: a new frontier in neonatal nursing. *Neonatal Nursing* **3**: 8–11.

Gorski, P.A., Hale, W. and Leonard, C. (1983) Direct computer recording of premature infants and nursing care: distress following two interventions. *Pediatrics* **72**: 198.

Gorski, P.A., Huntingdon, L. and Lewkowicz, D.J. (1990) Handling preterm infants in hospitals: stimulating controversy about timing of stimulation. *Clinics of Perinatology* **17**(1): 103–112.

Gottfried, A.W. and Gaiter, J.L. (1985) *Infant Stress Under Intensive Care: Environmental Neonatology.* Baltimore, Maryland: University Park Press.

Gottfried, A.W. and Hodgman, J. (1984) How intensive is newborn intensive care? An environmental analysis. *Pediatrics* **74**(2): 292–294.

Grunwald, P.C. and Becker, P.T. (1991) Developmental enhancement: implementing a program for the NICU. *Neonatal Network* **9**(6): 29–30, 39–45.

Gunderson, L.P. and Kenner, C. (1987) Neonatal stress: physiological adaptations and nursing implications. *Neonatal Network* **6**(1): 37–42.

Hallsworth, M. (1995) Positioning the pre-term infant. *Paediatric Nursing* **7**(1): 18–20.

Harrison, L.L. and Woods, S. (1991) Early parental touch and premature infants. *Journal of Obstetric, Gynecologic, and Neonatal Nursing* **20**(4): 299–306.

Harrison, L.L., Leeper, J.D. and Yoon, M. (1990) Effects of early parent touch on preterm infants' heart rates and arterial oxygen saturation levels. *Journal of Advanced Nursing* **15**: 877–885.

Harrison, L.L., Leeper, J.D. and Yoon, M. (1991) Preterm infants' physiologic responses to early parent touch. *Western Journal of Nursing Research* **13**(6): 698–713.

Hartelius, I. and Rasmussen, L. (1992) How little you are! *Neonatal Network* **11**(8): 33–40.

Hemingway, M.M. and Oliver, S.K. (1991) Water bed therapy and cranial moulding of the sick preterm infant. *Neonatal Network* **10**(3): 53–56.

Heriza, C.B. and Sweeney, J.K. (1990) Effects of NICU intervention on preterm infants: Part 2 — Implications for neonatal practice. *Infants and Young Children* **2**(3): 31–47.

Holditch-Davis, D. and Conway, A. (1992) Consent: Where research design meets reality. *Neonatal Network* **11**(4): 65–68.

Holditch-Davis, D. and Conway, A. (1993) Measuring the behaviour of high risk infants. *Neonatal Network* **12**(3): 69–72.

Horsley, A. (1990) The neonatal environment. *Paediatric Nursing* **February 1990**: 17–19.

Ingham, A. (1989) A review of the literature relating to touch and its use in intensive care. *Intensive Care Nursing* **5**: 65–75.

Isherwood, D. (1994) Baby massage groups. *Modern Midwife* **4**(2): 21–23.

Jorgensen, K.M. (1993) *Developmental Care of the Premature Infant: A Concise Overview*. S. Weymouth, USA: Developmental Care Division of Children's Medical Ventures.

Klaus, M.H. (1976) Bach, Beethoven or rock — and how much? *Journal of Pediatrics* **88**(2): 300.

Kling, P. (1989) Nursing interventions to decrease the risk of periventricular–intraventricular haemorrhage. *Journal of Obstetric, Gynecologic, and Neonatal Nursing* **18**(6): 457–464.

Koniak-Griffin, D. and Ludington-Hoe, S. (1988) Developmental and temperament outcomes of sensory stimulation in healthy infants. *Nursing Research* **32**(2): 70–76.

Korner, A.F. (1990) Infant stimulation: issues of theory and research. *Clinics in Perinatology* **17**(1): 173–183.

Kurlak, L.O., Ruggins, N.R. and Stephenson, T.J. (1994) Effect of nursing position on incidence, type and duration of clinically significant apnoea in preterm infants. *Archives of Disease in Childhood* **71**(1): 16–19.

Langer, V.S. (1990) Minimal handling protocol for the intensive care nursery. *Neonatal Network* **9**(3): 23–27.

Lawhon, G. and Melzar, A. (1988) Developmental care of the very low birth weight infant. *Journal of Perinatal–Neonatal Nursing* **2**(1): 56–65.

Leonard, J.E. (1993) Music therapy: fertile ground for application of research to practice. *Neonatal Network* **12**(2): 47–48.

Lester, B.M. and Tronick, E.Z. (1990) Introduction: Guidelines for stimulation with preterm infants. *Clinics in Perinatology* **17**(1): xv–xvii.

Letko, M.D. (1992) Detecting and preventing infant hearing loss. *Neonatal Network* **11**(5): 33–38.

Lioy, J. and Maginello, P. (1988) A comparison of prone and supine positioning in the immediate post extubation period of neonates. *Journal of Pediatrics* **112**: 982–984.

Lipsi, K., Clements-Shafer, K. and Hylton Rushton, C. (1991) Developmental rounds: an intervention strategy for hospitalized infants. *Pediatric Nursing* **17**(5): 433–437.

Long, J.G., Lucey, J.F. and Philip, A.G.S. (1980a) Noise and hypoxaemia in the intensive care nursery. *Pediatrics* **65**(1): 143–145.

Long, J.G., Philip, A.G.S. and Lucey, J.F. (1980b) Excessive handling as a cause of hypoxaemia. *Pediatrics* **65**(2): 203–207.

Lotas, M.J. (1992) Effects of light and sound in the neonatal intensive care unit environment on the low-birth-weight infant. *NAACOG's Clinical Issues in Perinatal and Women's Health Nursing* **3**(1): 34–44.

Lynch, M.E. (1991) Iatrogenic hazards, adverse occurrences, and complications involving NICU nursing practice. *Journal of Perinatal–Neonatal Nursing* **5**(3): 78–86.

McCain, G.C. (1992) Facilitating inactive awake states in preterm infants: a study of three interventions. *Nursing Research* **41**(3): 157–160.

McCormick, M.C. (1989) Long-term follow up of infants discharged from neonatal intensive care. *Journal of the American Medical Association* **261**: 1767–1772.

MacPhee, M. and Mori, C. (1991) Teaching nurses about neuromotor development: an evaluative study. *Pediatric Nursing* **17**(5): 438–444.

Mann, N.P., Haddow, R., Stokes, L., Goodley, S. and Rutter, N. (1986) Effect of night and day on preterm infants in a newborn nursery: randomised trial. *British Medical Journal* **293**(15): 1265–1267.

Mantovani, J.F. and Powers, J. (1991) Brain injury in premature infants: patterns on cranial ultrasound, their relationship to outcome, and the role of developmental intervention in the NICU. *Infants and Young Children* **4**(2): 20–32.

Marsden, D.J. (1980) Reduction of head flattening in preterm infants. *Developmental Medicine and Child Neurology* **22**: 507–509.

Masterson, J., Zucker, C. and Schulze, K. (1987) Prone and supine positioning effects on energy expenditure and behaviour of low birth weight neonates. *Pediatrics* **80**(5): 689–692.

Merenstein, G.B. and Gardner, S.L. (1993) *Handbook of Neonatal Intensive Care*, 3rd edn St. Louis, Missouri: Mosby-Year Book.

Miller, B.F. and Keane, C.B. (1983) *Encyclopedia and Dictionary of Medicine, Nursing and Allied Health*, 3rd edn Philadelphia, Pennsylvania: W.B. Saunders.

Mitchell, E.A. and Engelberts, A.C. (1991) Sleeping position and cot deaths. *Lancet* **338**: 192.

Munro, I. (1988) Prone or supine for preterm babies? *Lancet* **i** 688 (editorial).

Murdoch, D.R. and Darlow, B.A. (1984) Handling during neonatal intensive care. *Archives of Disease in Childhood* **59**: 957–961.

Nading, J.H. and Landes, R.D. (1984) Oxygen tension changes due to non-nutritive sucking (NNS) during orogastric tube feeding. *Pediatric Research* **18**(4): 206.

Nelson, D., Heitman, R. and Jennings, C. (1986) Effects of tactile stimulation on premature infant weight gain. *Journal of Obstetric, Gynecologic, and Neonatal Nursing* **15**(3): 262–267.

Norris, S., Campbell, L. and Brenkert, S. (1982) Nursing procedures and alterations in transcutaneous oxygen tension in premature infants. *Nursing Research* **31**(6): 330–336.

Oehler, J.M. (1993) Developmental care of low birth weight infants. *Nursing Clinics of North America* **28**(2): 289–301.

Oehler, J.M. and Cusson, R.M. (1994) Instrumentation in nursing research: commonly used statistics. *Neonatal Network* **13**(1): 63–65.

Oehler, J.M., Strickland, M. and Nordlund, C. (1991) Beyond technology: meeting developmental needs of infants in NICUs. *MCN; American Journal of Maternal Child Nursing* **16**(3): 148–151.

Page, J. and Cusson, R.M. (1993) Methodological issues: the

measurement of long term outcome. *Neonatal Network* **12**(7): 65–67.

Parker, A. (1990) Expert handling. *Nursing Times* **86**(12): 35–37.

Paterson, L. (1990) Baby massage in the neonatal unit. *Nursing* **4**(23): 19–21.

Perez-Woods, R. Malloy, M.B. and Tse, A.M. (1992) Positioning and skin care of the low-birth-weight neonate. *NAACOG's Clinical Issues in Perinatal and Women's Health* **3**(1): 97–113.

Perlman, J.M. and Volpe, J.J. (1983) Suctioning in the preterm infant: effects on cerebral blood flow velocity, intracranial pressure and arterial blood pressure. *Pediatrics* **72**(3): 329–334.

Peters, K.L. (1992) Does routine nursing care complicate the physiologic status of the premature neonate with respiratory distress syndrome? *Journal of Perinatal–Neonatal Nursing* **6**(2): 67–84.

Pickler, R.H. and Terrell, B.V. (1994) Non-nutritive sucking and necrotizing enterocolitis. *Neonatal Network* **13**(6): 15–18.

Pickler, R.H., Higgins, K.E. and Crummette, B.D. (1993) The effect of non-nutritive sucking on bottle-feeding stress in preterm infants. *Journal of Obstetric, Gynecologic, and Neonatal Nursing* **22**(3): 230–234.

Pym, S. (1992) *Positioning the Preterm Infant*. Bristol: Bristol Royal Hospital for Sick Children.

Resnick, M.B., Eyler, F.D., Nelson, R.M., Eitzman, D.V. and Bucciarelli, R.L. (1987) Developmental intervention for low birth weight infants: improved early developmental outcomes. *Pediatrics* **80**(1): 68–74.

Robinson, J., Moseley, M. and Fielder, A. (1990) Illuminance of neonatal units. *Archives of Disease in Childhood* **65**: 679–682.

Romanko, M.V. and Bost, B.A. (1982) Swaddling: an effective intervention for pacifying infants. *Pediatric Nursing* **8**(4): 259–261.

Russell, J. (1993) Touch and infant massage. *Paediatric Nursing* **5**(3): 8, 10–11.

Sayre-Adams, J. (1991) Therapeutic touch. *Nursing Standard* **5**(45): 28.

Sehgal, S.K., Prakash, O., Gupta, A., Mohan, M. and Anand, N.K. (1990) Evaluation of beneficial effects of non-nutritive sucking in preterm infants. *Indian Pediatrics* **27**: 263–266.

Shultz, C.M. (1992) Nursing roles: optimizing premature infant outcomes. *Neonatal Network* **11**(3): 9–13.

Simbruner, G., Coradello, H., Fodor, H., Havelec, L., Lubec, G. and Pollak, A. (1981) Effect of tracheal suction on oxygenation, circulation and lung mechanics in the newborn infant. *Archives of Disease in Childhood* **56**: 326–330.

Sisson, T.R.C. (1985) Hazards to vision in the nursery. *New England Journal of Medicine* **313**(7): 444–445.

Slusher, I.L. and McClure, M.J. (1992) Infant stimulation during hospitalization. *Journal of Paediatric Nursing* **7**(4): 276–279.

Sparshott, M. (1990) The human touch. *Paediatric Nursing* **2**(5): 8–10.

Sparshott, M. (1991) Reducing infant trauma. *Nursing Times* **87**(50): 30–32.

Speidel, B.D. (1978) Adverse effects of routine procedures on preterm infants. *Lancet* **1**: 864–866.

Stewart Hegedus, K.S. and Madden, J.E. (1994) Caring in a neonatal intensive care unit: perspectives of providers and consumers. *Journal of Perinatal–Neonatal Nursing* **8**(2): 67–75.

Strauch, C., Brandt, S. and Edwards-Beckett, J. (1993) Implementation of a quiet hour: effect on noise levels and infant sleep states. *Neonatal Network* **12**(2): 31–35.

Szabo, J.S., Hillemeir, A.C. and Oh, W. (1985) Effect of non-nutritive and nutritive suck on gastric emptying in preterm infants. *Journal of Pediatric Gastroenterology and Nutrition* **4**(3): 348–351.

Thomas, K.A. and Conway, A. (1991) Multi-site studies. *Neonatal Network* **10**(3): 74–75.

Thomas, K.A. and Conway, A. (1992) Validity: controlling for variables in research studies involving high risk neonates. *Neonatal Network* **11**(6): 97–100.

Treas, L.S. (1993) Incubator covers: health or hazard? *Neonatal Network* **12**(8): 50–51.

Tribotti, S.J. and Stein, M. (1992) From research to clinical practice: implementing the NIDCAP. *Neonatal Network* **11**(2): 35–40.

Tronick, E.Z., Scanlon, K.B. and Scanlon, J.W. (1990) Protective apathy, a hypothesis about the behavioural organization and its relation to clinical and physiologic status of the preterm infant during the newborn period. *Clinics in Perinatology* **17**(1): 125–154.

Tucker Catlett, A. and Holditch-Davis, D. (1990) Environmental stimulation of the acutely ill premature infant: physiological effects and nursing implications. *Neonatal Network* **8**(6): 19–25.

Tudehope, D.I and Thearle, M.J. (1989) *A Primer of Neonatal Medicine*, 2nd edn. Brisbane: Brooks Waterloo.

Turrill, J. (1992) Supported positioning in intensive care. *Paediatric Nursing* **4**(4): 24–27.

United Kingdom Central Council For Nursing, Midwifery and Health Visiting (1992) *Code of Professional Conduct*. London: UKCC.

Updike, C., Schmidt, R.E., Macke, C., Cahoon, J. and Miller, M. (1986) Positional support for premature infants. *American Journal of Occupational Therapy* **40**(10): 712–715.

Vandenberg, K.A. (1985) Revising the traditional model: an individualized approach to developmental interventions in the intensive care nursery. *Neonatal Network* **3**(5): 32–38.

Warren, I. (1993) How to place a baby. *MIDIRS Midwifery Digest* **3**(4): 452–453.

Weber, K.M. (1991) Massage for stressed infants. *International Journal of Alternative and Complementary Medicine* **9**(12): 9–10.

Weibley, T.T. (1989) Inside the incubator. *MCN; American Journal of Maternal Child Health Nursing* **14**: 996–100.

Werner, N.P. and Conway, A.E. (1990) Caregiver contacts experienced by premature infants in the neonatal intensive care unit. *Maternal–Child Nursing Journal* **19**(11): 21–43.

White-Traut, R.C. and Goldman, M.B.C. (1988) Premature infant massage: is it safe? *Pediatric Nursing* **14**(4): 285–289.

White-Traut, R.C. and Hutchens Pate, C.M.H. (1987) Modulating infant state in premature infants. *Journal of Pediatric Nursing* **2**(2): 96–101.

White-Traut, R.C., Silvestri, J.M., Nelson, M.N., Patel, M.K. and Kilgallon, D. (1993) Patterns of physiologic and behavioural response of intermediate care preterm infants to intervention. *Pediatric Nursing* **19**(6): 625–629.

Whitley, S. and Cowan, M. (1991) Developmental intervention in the newborn intensive care unit. *NAACOG's Clinical Issues in Perinatal and Women's Health Nursing* **2**(1): 84–110.

Wigfield, R.E., Fleming, P.J., Berry, P.J., Rudd, P.T. and Golding, J. (1992) Can the fall in Avon's sudden infant death rate be explained by changes in sleeping position. *British Medical Journal* **304**: 282–283.

Wolke, D. (1987) Environmental neonatology. *Archives of Disease in Childhood* **62**: 987–988.

Woodson, R. and Hamilton, C. (1988) The effects of non-nutritive sucking on heart rate in preterm infants. *Developmental Psychobiology* **21**(3): 207–213.

Woodson, R., Drinkwin, J. and Hamilton, C. (1985) Effects of non-nutritive sucking on state and activity: term–preterm comparisons. *Infant Behaviour and Development* **8**(4): 435–441.

Wright Lott, J. (1989) Developmental care of the preterm infant. *Neonatal Network* **7**(4): 21–28.

Yecco, G.J. (1993) Neurobehavioural development and developmental support of premature infants. *Journal of Perinatal–Neonatal Nursing* **7**(1): 56–65.

Young, J. (1994) Nursing preterm babies in intensive care: which position is best? *JNN: Journal of Neonatal Nursing* **1**(1): 27–31.

Young, V. (1995) *Tools for Living—Prem Positioners*. Uxbridge: Brunel Institute for Bioengineering, Brunel University.

Bibliography

Ayres, A.J. (1989) *Sensory Integration and the Child*. Los Angeles, California: Western Psychological Services.

Brink, P.J. and Wood, M.J. (1989) *Advanced Design in Nursing Research*. Newbury Park, California: Sage Publications.

British Standards Institution (1989) *British Standard Recommendations for References to Published Materials, BS1629: 1989*. UK: Information and Documentation Standards Policy Committee, British Standards Institution.

Guralnick, M.J. and Bennett, F.C. (eds) (1987). *The Effectiveness of Early Intervention for At-Risk and Handicapped Children*. London: Academic Press.

Hannon, K.M. (1993) Support can reduce the stress factor: stress in neonatal nursing. *Professional Nurse* **8**(8): 496, 498, 500.

Morrison, P. (1991) Critiquing research. *Surgical Nurse* **4**(3): 20–22.

Nugent, K. (1989) Routine care: promoting development in hospitalized infants. *MCN; American Journal of Maternal Child Nursing*: **14**(5): 318.

Sweeney, J. (ed.) (1986) *The High-Risk Neonate: Developmental Therapy Perspectives*. New York: Haworth Press.

Tatano-Beck, C. (1990) The research critique: general criteria for evaluating a research report. *Journal of Obstetric, Gynecologic, and Neonatal Nursing* **19**(1): 18–22.

Treece, E.W. and Treece, J.W. (1986) *Elements of Research in Nursing*, 4th edn. St Louis, Missouri: C.V. Mosby.

Turabian, K.L. (1987) *A Manual for Writers of Term Papers, Theses, and Dissertations*, 5th edn. Chicago, Illinois: University of Chicago Press.

Useful Addresses

Bettacare Ltd
Bettacare House
9/10 Faygate Business Centre
Faygate
West Sussex RH12 4DN
UK

Tel 01293-851 896
Fax 01293-851 065

Children's Medical Ventures
541 Main Street
Suite 416, S.Weymouth
MA 02190
USA

Fax 617-337-5938

Monin-Orthopedie Fabricant
186 Rue du Faubourg Saint-Martin
75010 Paris
France

Tel 16(1) 46 07 59 41
Fax 16(1) 42 05 61 45

Neonatal Positioning Project
Vivien Young
'Tools for Living'
Brunel Institute for Bioengineering
Brunel University
Uxbridge
Middlesex UB8 3PH
UK

Tel 01895-271 206
Fax 01895-274 608

Scan Mobility Ltd
Lasal Rehab
St Martin's House
St Martin's in the Field
Altcar Lane
Formby L37 6AJ
UK

Tel 01704-834 483
Fax 01704-834 484

Sew Soft
Babynest
C/o Stephanie Dyer
Boncath Uchaf
Dyfed SA37 0HR
UK
Tel 01239-841 712

Tarry Manufacturing
16 East Franklin Street
Danbury
CT 06810
USA

Tel 203-794-1438
Fax 203-792-5581

Vickers Medical
Ruxley Corner
Sidcup
Kent DA14 5BL
UK

Tel 0181-309 0433
Fax 0181-309 0919

Index